D0793574

# The Springer Series on Death and Suicide

ROBERT KASTENBAUM, Ph.D., Series Editor

*Dame Cicely Saunders, O. M., D. B. E., F. R. C. P.*, is the founder and guiding spirit of the international hospice care movement. She has been awarded The Order of Merit by the Queen of England and more than twenty honorary degrees from universities in the United States and the United Kingdom, along with the British Medical Association's Gold Medal. Under her leadership, St. Christopher's Hospice (Sydenham, London) has become the pre-eminent model for hospice research and training as well as service. Dame Saunders is author of *The Management of Terminal Malignant Disease* and many other publications that are central to the provision of palliative care throughout the world

*Robert Kastenbaum, Ph.D.*, is Professor of Gerontology in the Department of Communication, Arizona State University. A clinician, researcher, dramatist, and educator, he served as consultant to The National Hospice Demonstration Project, and has received awards as outstanding death educator from the Association of Death Education and Counseling and the National Center for Death Education. His books include *The Psychology of Death* and *Death, Society, and Human Experience*. He is editor of *Omega, Journal of Death and Dying*.

# Hospice Care
# on the
# International Scene

Dame Cicely Saunders, OM, DBE, FRCP
Robert Kastenbaum, PhD
Editors

Springer Publishing Company

Copyright © 1997 by Springer Publishing Company, Inc.

Springer Publishing Company, Inc.
536 Broadway
New York, NY 10012-3955

Cover design by Margaret Dunin
Production Editor: Kathleen Kelly

97 98 99 00 01/5 4 3 2 1

Library of Congress Cataloging-in-Publication Data

Hospice care on the international scene/Dame Cicely Saunders, Robert
    Kastenbaum, editors.
        p.   cm.—(Springer series on death and suicide)
    Includes bibliographical references and index.
    ISBN 0-8261-9580-6
    1. Hospices.   2. Hospice care.   I. Saunders, Cicely M., Dame.
II. Kastenbaum, Robert.   III. Series.
RA1000.H67   1997
362.1'756—dc21                                          96-40364
                                                            CIP

Printed in the United States of America

# Contents

v

# Foreword

The world's catalog of sorrows and tragedies has continued to lengthen in recent years. Many lives are in jeopardy in many places, even as these words are being written. Nevertheless, the human spirit has not remained passive and helpless. The ongoing development of palliative care programs for terminally ill people provides one of the most significant and encouraging examples of effective response to circumstances that threaten core human values.

This book tells part of the story. The part it tells is perhaps the part that most needs telling at this time: how hospice care has been taking root throughout much of the world, and how dedicated and open-minded people are finding ways to shape hospice care to the particular needs and resources of their countries and communities. Much of the professional and general public literature describing hospice programs has been derived from programs in the United Kingdom and North America. Only occasionally are there reminders that the relief of suffering is a universal concern and that efforts are being made in the rural areas of developing countries as well as the urban centers of the Western world.

Who can tell this story better than the people who are engaged in the process of establishing, securing, and expanding palliative care programs throughout the world? We have called upon many of these people, and they have responded most generously with their time and effort. We are grateful to contributors from all over the globe who voluntarily added to their demanding everyday responsibilities the effort required to write a chapter or complete a detailed questionnaire.

The story is told in two ways. Most of this book consists of chapters that describe either a specific hospice program or the overall development of palliative care in a country. This division is not rigorous, because the story of a particular hospice often reveals the broader picture of an entire nation's struggle to bring palliative care to those in need. Included here are reports from pioneering hospice programs in Asia, the Middle East, tropical Africa, and a country under the

Communist regime, as well as many other programs that represented striking departures from the pollicies and practices of the homeland.

Contributing authors were asked to describe the origins and subsequent development of their palliative programs—conflicts, frustrations, and mistakes included. They were invited to help the reader see the problems, issues, and choices through the eyes of the people who were attempting to make hospice care a reality in their land. We also asked the contributors to look ahead. What problems have yet to be solved? What plans have yet to be actualized? Some of the contributing authors have made numerous contributions to the literature; others were writing their first manuscript for professional publication. All have told their stories with the authenticity of their personal experiences, some in a remarkably concise manner, others at greater length. Taken together, these contributions describe hospice programs in all major regions of the globe. There are some unfortunate gaps in coverage of particular countries for various reasons, primarily the pressure of operational responsibilities that prevented some programs from contributing chapters within the available time frame. We hope additional voices will be heard in the future.

The presentations have an archival value. They will serve as a record of how the international hospice movement functioned during the critical early period. More significantly, however, these presentations have an immediate value to all who are concerned with the humane and effective care of terminally ill people and their families. It is one of the striking characteristics of the international hospice care movement that the participants are eager to learn from each other. This learning process was at first primarily unidirectional, as experts in the United Kingdom shared their knowledge and imparted their skills to others. Now, however, and in the future, the learning process has become omnidirectional. We can all learn from the experiences and achievements of hospice workers throughout the world.

The story has also been told through numbers. A questionnaire was sent to all programs listed in the files of St. Christopher's Hospice Information Service. Completed questionnaires were received from 103 programs in 31 countries. Basic findings are presented to provide an overview that supplements the individual hospice and national reports.

The book begins with a hospice mission statement by Dame Cicely Saunders and concludes with a brief review and commentary by the coeditors. In between these entry and exit chapters we think you will find facts, ideas, and experiences that enhance understanding of hospice care on the international scene.

# Contributors

**Dr. Avis Boyar,**
Oncology Department MBC 64
King Faisal Specialist Hospital and Research
Centre
P. O. Box 3354 Riyadh 11211
Saudi Arabia

**Peter Buckland,**
Executive Dirctor
Hospice of Southern Africa
P. O. Box 38785
Pinelands 7430
Republic of South Africa

**G. L. Burn,**
St. Christopher's Hospice
51-59 Lawrie Park Road
Sydenham
London SE26 6DZ
England

**Lucy S. T. Chung,**
Nursing Director
Bradbury Hospice, A Kung Kok
Shan Road, Shatin
Hong Kong

**Giovanni Creton, M.D.**
Medical Director
Ryder Italia
Viale Romania 32
00197 Rome, Italy

**Dr. Isa de Jaramillo,**
Clinical Psychologist
Fundacion Omega,
Dra. F #119-14 Cors 408
Bogota, Colombia

**Ann Eve**
St. Christopher's Hospice
51-59 Lawrie Park Road
Sydenham
London SE26 6DZ
England

**Dr. Adnan Ezzat,**
Oncology Department MBC 64
King Faisal Specialist Hospital and Research
Centre
P. O. Box 3354 Riyadh 11211
Saudi Arabia

**Ann Smith Gordon, RN, JP,**
President and Chief Executive Officer
Patients Assitance League and Service
P.O. Box DV19
Devonshire DV BX Bermuda

**Alan J. Gray, M. B.. Ch. B. FRACP, FRACR,**
Palliative Care Physician
Oncology Department MBC 64
King Faisal Specialist Hospital and Research
Centre
P. O. Box 3354 Riyadh 11211
Saudi Arabia

**Virginia-Ann Gumley**
St. Christopher's Hospice
51-59 Lawrie Park Road
Sydenham
London SE26 6DZ
England

**Dr. Rana Hammad,**
Director,
Al-Malath Foundation for Humanistic Care
P.O. Box 85136
Amman 11185
Jordan

**Joan Hunt,**
President
Dra. Marisa Martin Rosello
CUDECA
Ed. Gavilan. Puebla Lucia
Fuengirola, Malaga
Spain 29640

**Avril Jackson**
St. Christopher's Hospice
51-59 Lawrie Park Road
Sydenham
London SE26 6DZ
England

**Dr. Malcolm Joblin & Staff**
Cranford Hawke's Bay Hospice
P.O. Box 89119
Havelock North, New Zealand

**Anica Jusic, President,**
Croatian Society for Hospice/Palliative Care
Gunrhuliceva 49/I
Zagreb, Croatia 10,000

**Robert Kastenbaum, Ph.D**
Arizona State Univesity
Department of Communication
Box 871205
Tempe, Arizona 85287-1205.

**D. McElvaine,**
Senior Administrator,
Island Hosice Service
60 Livingstone Avenue
P.O. Box CV 7
Causeway, Harare, Zimbabwe

**Balfour Mount, M.D.**
687 Pine Ave West
Montreal Quebec
H3A 1A1 Canada

**Mitsuaki Sakonji, M.D.**
Jizankai Medical Foundation Tsuboi Cancer
Center Hospital
1-10-13, Asakamachi, Nagakubo
Kohriyama-she, Fukushima
Japan 963-01

**Dr. Michele H. Salamagne**
Medical Director
Unite de Soins Palliatif
Hospital Paul Brousse
14 av. Paul Vaillant Coururier
Villejuif Cedex 94804
France

**Dame Cicely Saunders, OM, DBE, FRCP,**
Chairman, St. Christopher's Hospice
51-59 Lawrie Park Road
Sydenham
London SE26 6DZ
England

**Chise Shimizu**
Jizankai Medical Foundation Tsuboi Cancer
Center Hospital
1-10-13, Asakamachi, Nagakubo
Kohriyama-she, Fukushima
Japan 963-01

**Yae Shinjo**
Jizankai Medical Foundation Tsuboi Cancer
Center Hospital
1-10-13, Asakamachi, Nagakubo
Kohriyama-she, Fukushima
Japan 963-01

**Dr. Anthony Smith**
Gillmead, Rutland Gate
Bromley Kent
BR2 0TG
United Kingdom

**Jan Stjernsward, MD, Ph.D., Chief**
Cancer and Palliative Care Unit
World Health Organization
CH-1211 Geneva 27 Switzerland

**Janina Jujawska Tenner, M.D.**
Zakatek 7/64
Krakow Poland 30076

**Eitaka Tsuboi, M.D.**
Jizankai Medical Foundation Tsuboi Cancer
Center Hospital
1-10-13, Asakamachi, Nagakubo
Kohriyama-she, Fukushima
Japan 963-01

**Alexander Waller, M.D.**
Acting Medical Director
Tel Hashomer Hospice
Building 32, Sheba Medical Centra
Tel Hashomer, Israel

**Marilyn Wilson, M.A.**
Arizona State University
Department of Communication
Box 871205
Tempe, Arizona 85287-1205

**Dr. Douglas Zuefu Zhu, M.D.**
1214 31st Street, Apt. 3A
Des Moines, Iowa 50311

# PART I

## Introduction to the International Hospice Movement

---

# Hospices Worldwide: A Mission Statement

## Dame Cicely Saunders

It has been said that people tend to be either "woodcutters" or "planters." Some clear the ground for future development; others till the soil and sow and harvest the crop. The commitment and skills of both groups has been called on in the development of modern hospice principles and techniques. The contributors to this book illustrate this process in describing the way hospice care is establishing itself throughout much of the world.

The need for such a movement was clearly articulated by Patrick Wall (1986):

> Up to the 19th century, most medical care related to the amelioration of symptoms, while the natural history of the disease took its course towards recovery or death. By 1900 doctors and patients alike had turned to a search for root cause and ultimate cure. In the course of this new direction, symptoms were placed on one side as signposts along a highway which was being driven towards the intended direction. Therapies directed at the signposts were denigrated . . . as merely symptomatic. By the second half of this century, a reaction had set in as is seen by such remarkable developments as the hospice movement. The immediate origins of misery and suffering need immediate attention, while the long-term search for basic cure proceeds. The old methods of care and caring had to be rediscovered and the best of modern medicine had to be turned to the task of new study and therapy, specifically directed at pain. (p. 1)

Both care and skill were asked for by David Tasma, the 40-year-old Jewish patient from Warsaw whom I met in 1947. The real founder of St. Christopher's Hospice, he said, "I want what is in your mind and in your heart." This commission led, on reflection, to the realization that patients facing the end of life, as he was, would need all the skills that could be developed, researched, and taught—together with the friendship and care of the heart. He felt that he had done nothing in his life for the world to remember, but his gesture in leaving me five hundred pounds in his will "to be a window in your Home" was the beginning of this worldwide movement. The "Home" he referred to was something we had discussed together, a place where people would have the space and openness so hard to come by in a busy surgical ward. His use of the word "window" led me to understand that we should be open to the world, to all who would come—patients, families, and those who wanted to learn. Later I extended this to an openness among ourselves and, finally, to the beyond. This sharing has continued to grow over the years.

After his quiet death, I finally felt assured that he had made his own journey, looking to the faith of his fathers after many years of agnosticism. He had made this journey in a complete freedom of the spirit. Hospice has therefore adopted these principles: openness, mind together with heart, and deep concern for the freedom of each individual to make his or her own journey toward their goals.

David Tasma died in February, 1948, and I immediately enrolled as a volunteer nurse in one of the established homes for terminal care. St. Luke's Hospital (originally "The Home for the Dying Poor") had been opened in London in 1893. After 3 years I had planned to leave my post as a medical social worker and return somehow to nursing in his field (palliative care) (my career as a registered nurse having been interrupted by problems with my back). The surgeon for whom I was working thought otherwise and said: "Go and read medicine. It's the doctors who desert the dying. There is so much more to learned about pain and you will only be frustrated if you don't do it properly—and they won't listen to you."

Supported financially by my father and helped by Mr. Barrett, the surgeon, I enrolled in medical training. I continued as a nurse volunteer for another 4 years and observed the regular giving of oral opiates, which provided much better pain relief than I had seen in my earlier roles at a London teaching hospital. But above all, I spent my time listening to patients.

The next step in a "woodcutting" career sent me to St. Joseph's Hospice (founded in 1905) on a clinical research fellowship. Virtually untouched by medical advances, the infinitely caring nuns welcomed a doctor who was prepared to introduce drug sheets, patients' notes and reports, and took the time to listen. Insteading of "earning" their morphine by suffering pain first, the patients were offered relief on a regular basis. We took the drugs they were already receiving on an "as required" basis and introduced a regular routine that, when individually adjusted, prevents pain from constantly recurring. Patients were freed from the cycle in which their experiences alternated between "pain-full to pain-free," as one of the nuns recalls it. This practice was soon extended to an analysis and treatment of symptoms "which I watched (helplessly) until you came on the scene," as the same nun wrote recently to me.

The presentation of this work in a series of six articles in the *Nursing Times* in 1959 coincided with the publication of Herman Feifel's *The Meaning of Death,* Rene Fox's *Experiment Perilous,* and the foundation of Cruse (an organization for widows) in London. The first of many lectures on the nature and management of terminal pain was given in the Royal Society of Medicine in the winter of 1962 and published the next year, as I neared the end of a survey of the work at St. Joseph's from 1,100 case notes.

The first trip to the U. S. in 1963 took place when a steering group registered St. Christopher's Hospice as a charity. "Hospice means help for travellers? Well, you will have to have St. Christopher, won't you?" said a patient I was caring for, one of the many who were deeply involved in these plans for a modern research and teaching hospice. These patients were the *real* fundraisers, as well as the inspiration for the principles of hospice that are now interpreted around the world. This work also led to palliative medicine being recognized as a new medical specialty in the United Kingdom in 1987.

## BASIC PRINCIPLES OF HOSPICE CARE

The three basic tenets given by the experience with David Tasma in 1948 had, by St. Christopher's opening in 1967, led to a set of principles which have stood the test of time and reinterpretation in a great variety of cultures. These are:

1) *The skilled analysis of pain and symptom control, presented as Total Pain.* As one patient remembered:

> Well, doctor, it began in my back but now it seems that all of me is wrong. I could have cried for the pills and the injections but I knew that I must not. Nobody seems to understand and I felt as if all the world was against me. My husband and son were marvellous, but they were having to stay off work and lose their wages. But it's so marvellous to start feeling safe again.

Here, physical, mental, social, and spiritual pain are all described in the answer to one question: "Mrs. H., tell me about your pain." The patient's whole experience of pain has been the basis for numerous lectures and articles presented over the intervening years. This basically simple system has been translated into many languages and widely distributed by the World Health Organization in a booklet entitled *Cancer Pain Relief,* first published in 1986. Its three-step ladder of nonopioids, weak opioids, and strong opioids, all with appropriate adjuvants, is now widely known. The status bestowed by its WHO endorsement has been used to impel governments to legalize possibilities of pain relief that had often been unobtainable or hedged about with restrictions in many parts of the world.

2) *Input from a multidisciplinary team is needed to relieve the experience of total pain and enable a person to face what is happening in his or her individual way. This relief should be available whether the person is at home, hospice, or hospital, in space freed from the presence or threat of pain, breathlessness, and other forms of suffering.*

Other specialties work in this cooperative way. The need for such cooperation is especially important when dealing with a crisis situation in which a person faces the "many-headed dragon" of total pain. A medieval picture of such a dragon was given to me by a patient. "That's what my illness feels like to me," she said. Another patient drew a singleheaded dragon with the same interpretation. In this picture, the dragon confronted a small child. The dragon was eating the flowers scattered at her feet, but the child was not afraid. "Sometimes the dragon holds the treasure," as one of our consults put it, reminding us of many myths and fairy tales.

3) *To maximize the potential remaining to a patient or family, not only in quality of physical ease but also in relationships and the possibilities of turning toward their own inner values.*

As St. Christopher's Mission Statement puts it, palliative care exists not only to affirm life and individuality, but also "to help patients with strong and unfamiliar emotions, to assist them to explore meaning, purpose, and value in their lives. To offer opportunity to reconcile and heal relationships and complete important personal tasks."

4) *The whole "family," whatever its nature, is the focus and unit of care (and frequently the caring team) both during and after the patient's illness and in bereavement.*

Much has been learned over the years in different countries, but whatever the culture, a hospice team tries to help families find again the strengths that have helped them through other adversities. This time of crisis often leads to new growth and creativity. It is a moment of truth for them as well as for the patient, a truth sometimes in silent meeting rather than in words.

5) *Helping the dying is a taxing task for a single person, although some have changed the whole climate of a hospital by their skill and diplomacy. Most of us need the support of working in a team, and peer groups should be ready to assist each other to come to terms with the emotional anguish they must expect to encounter.*

Additionally, administration must be flexible and approachable, ready to knit volunteers and professionals together, each confident in their own roles. Hospice teams tend to grow together as a community united by their common aim.

6) *Recording, analysis, and appropriate research have enabled palliative care to be accepted in a variety of settings.* The initial focus on pain in cancer and also in motor neurone disease (amyotrophic lateral sclerosis, "Lou Gehrig's disease") has enabled many well-recognized studies to be undertaken in all branches of this multifaceted work.

Publication in general as well as in specialist journals has been the objective foundation of a widespread program of education and sharing with people in all disciplines. The early experience at St. Joseph's has been expanded by the work of other pioneers in this field to establish a sound body of expertise, with a willingness to solve new problems or look again at accepted wisdom. Hospice work is not to be regarded as a soft option, but as a specialty that combines scientific rigor with compassion.

7) *The search for meaning is not only a challenge of patients and families. As individuals and as a caring team, many workers feel compelled to seek answers or, more often, to develop a readiness to live with questions.*

Many teams include people with a religious commitment, but the original challenge to openness has meant that most groups form a community of the unlike. Above all, their questionings and answers must never be imposed on patients. We aim to give patients space in a climate that offers hope and even expectation. They are to sing their own song, not that of the palliative care team. The chaplaincy at St. Christopher's includes a researcher who is working on a project entitled, "A Search for Sources of Meaning and Sense of Self in Dying People." The indifferent and the atheist have their welcome and place among us.

A group from St. Christopher's started discussing these issues 5 years before the Hospice opened. Its original aim and basis was recently expressed in a shortened form as follows:

- St. Christopher's Hospice is committed to giving the best possible palliative care to the terminally ill, both in the hospice and in home care. It encourages a freedom of expression and belief and affirms the sacredness of each individual and the range of individual needs in the final days of their human journey.
- St. Christopher's welcomes the practice of those of all faiths and recognizes the value of the contribution to its objectives by those of any faith or none.
- St. Christopher's was established and has grown as a Christian foundation, not simply in terms of its care but from a belief that the God revealed in

Christ shared and shares the darkness of suffering and dying and has transformed the reality of death.

- The wider spiritual dimension at St. Christopher's has been built up from the creativity and growth of many of its patients and witnesses to the discovery of their own strengths by countless families; it has also developed through the experiences of its staff, a community of the unlike.

It is also appropriate to reprint here a paper I drew up with help from St. Christopher's team in 1976, and which has been recently reprinted in our *Hospice Bulletin*. It was the foundation of the work of our Hospice Information Service. I am prepared to stand by this document as a whole after 20 additional years of work and development.

## ESSENTIALS FOR A HOSPICE*

## A. Planning

1. This work should not be embarked on unless you really cannot help it, i.e., someone, preferably a doctor, must be prepared to be a leader, have an over-powering desire to get it going, and be prepared to sweat and pray to do this.
2. It must be autonomous, with control over the selection of its patients and staff. If it is part of a large complex it will need a fairly powerful leader/ director to ensure this.
3. It must be medically respectable, giving care which will demand attention and in due course cooperation from those outside. Discussion with doctors locally should start at an early stage.
4. A home care program should be planned from the start. This means the area served, transportation, and so forth must be researched and the local community, especially the family doctors, informed and involved.
5. Get the support of the National Health Service (or equivalent) in principle, and early, but if possible have some independence as control over your own policy is essential.
6. It should be small., e.g., 50–70 beds *maximum*. Most will be much smaller but should be large enough to give the best quality medical, nursing, paramedical and administrative practice. This should include home care.
7. The building should be attractive; purpose-built if possible. Good transportation for visitors is essential.

* Reprinted from

8. Select your architects, preferably with experience in this field, as early as possible. Invite them to your preliminary discussions where they should be able to help with your brief. Some of your enthusiasm may well rub off on them.

9. It must not be thought of as a place "only for the dying." There must be some kind of mixture of patients, e.g., including long-stay and those to be discharged after pain control, to help relationships with the surrounding community.

10. Go around and see what is being done, and then see how your own circumstances can produce another version. There is need for diversity in this field.

## B. Working

11. You should accept the demand and need to teach, and must look at what you are doing on an objective basis. Add research when and where you can.

12. Plan, teach, and act on the assumption that the patient's family is part of the unit of care as well as being part of the care-giving team. Concern for their well-being does not end with the patient's death.

13. The relief or prevention of pain and other sources of physical and emotional distress is the pivot of the work and requires continuous monitoring of responses to drugs and other interventions, together with a stubborn reluctance to accept defeat.

14. High staff ratio for nurses, so people can give time. Be prepared to train your own auxiliaries and to welcome people back to nursing. Do all possible to support a stable staff. For this we suggest:

    i)    One or two seniors must have had experience in this work.
    ii)   Put emphasis on team work, conversations, and support.
    iii)  Create your own patchwork of whole- and part-timers.
    iv)   Be prepared to employ the unlikely but not the unstable.
    v)    Avoid people working out their own bereavements too soon.
    vi)   Have a play group and school social club for children of the staff.
    vii)  Remember that all staff need support.
    viii) Learn how to garner and use volunteers from the local community as part of the team. Get into contact with them (and many of your staff) through local church and other groups.

15. Good spiritual care is essential to support your staff as well as patients. This cannot be grafted on unless there is some kind of religious foundation from the beginning.

16. Hospice work seems to need the kind of conviction that is prepared to go on asking questions, has no rigid answers, but has an overall confidence that there is meaning and an answer, even if it is not yet revealed.

17. The group must be prepared to meet together, have parties and social occasions but, above all, pray. There must not be a dogmatic line but there must be an agreed attitude, and some sense of help coming from beyond the individuals and the group. Everyone must have thought about the question, "Where do you go when you are desperate?"

18. As far as possible the hospice must be so flexible that you can respect the frame of reference of each individual patient, allowing him/her to guide what is done, consciously or unconsciously, never feeling a burden and assured that the family will be all right, both during his/her stay in the hospice and afterwards.

19. To do this, there must be open communication in all directions among the staff. Although there must be proper responsibility and authority, no one should hide behind a hierarchy and people should work together in a way which will enable a community to grow. Community is a gift to people who really work together.


## A REMARKABLE SPREAD OF SKILL AND CARE

During the two decades that have passed since this document was drawn up, innumerable people across the world have started out in their own ways, responding to the need they have seen around them. Many have set up outside their particular health care system. Others have worked within the existing system. This book describes diverse groups, all with the desire that patients and families should find relief and dignity at the end of life. All of us in this demanding and rewarding field find our way by listening to people in need and by recognizing the achievements they so often bring out of their adversity.

Although much of the network of palliative care in the United Kingdom has included inpatient hospices, some five times as many people are supported as a complimentary local service at home by St. Christopher's staff. This figure is estimated to apply across the country as a whole. Since St. Christopher's pioneered home care in 1969, numbers have escalated, and it seems likely that this will continue to increase to match the demand. Home care is the pattern in most other countries. At the same time, however, palliative medicine is being introduced into many hospitals. Both these developments are bringing hospice attitudes and skills into mainstream medicine, and new and imaginative plans are constantly being developed.

The years since David Tasma died have seen a remarkable spread of skill and care. At the same time, however, there has been an increasing demand for the legalization of physician-assisted suicide and active, voluntary euthanasia. Palliative care offers an alternative approach between this move and the compulsion to press active "curative" treatment, however inappropriate. The palliative approach should not be limited to special teams and particular diagnoses, but should be spread widely.

The line between voluntary and involuntary euthanasia will be impossible to maintain, according to a recent House of Lords Select Committee Report on Medical Ethics (1994). The New York Task Force on Life and the Law also states:

> Recent proposals to legalize assisted suicide and euthanasia in some states would transform the right to decide about medical treatment into a far broader right to control the timing and manner of death. After lengthy deliberations, the Task Force unanimously concluded that the dangers of such a dramatic change in public policy would far outweigh any possible benefits. In light of the pervasive failure of our health care system to treat pain and diagnose and treat depression, legalizing assisted suicide and euthanasia would be profoundly dangerous for many individuals who are ill and vulnerable. The risks would be most severe for those who are elderly, poor, socially disadvantaged, or without access to good medical care. Members of the Task Force hold different views about the ethical acceptability of assisted suicide and euthanasia. Despite these differences, they unanimously recommend that existing law should not be changed to permit these practices (New York State Task Force on Life and the Law 1994).

Support at home is the first choice for most people around the world. However, Hinton's detailed study (1994) showed that where hospice beds were available, realistic preference for home care fell steadily from 100% to 54% of patients and 45% of relatives. The availability of backup beds in St. Christopher's has often enabled families to carry on longer than they expected, knowing that much needed relief was at hand. In many parts of the world, this is not so, nor are comparatively expensive buildings likely to become available. The thrust now is surely both to increase the teaching of families at home and staff in hospitals, and to show what can be done once effective symptom control is established.

Centers will still be needed for research and teaching, but the local groups described in this book are as much the future as the growing number of national and international associations. The heart of hospice has always been the open contacts between people, the offer of friendship together with skill, and the support of the freedom of the spirit for everyone, whatever their circumstances.

# REFERENCES

Feifel, H. (Ed.) (1959). *The meaning of death.* New York: McGraw-Hill.
Fox, R. (1959). *Experiment perilous.* Glencoe, IL: The Free Press.

Hinton, J. (1994). Can home care maintain an acceptable quality of life for patients with terminal cancer and their relatives? *Palliative Medicine, 8,* 183–196.

Official Statement. (1994). New York advises on assisted suicide. *Bulletin of Medical Ethics,* 8–11.

Wall, P. D. (1986). Editorial: 25 volumes of *Pain. Pain, 25,* 1–4.

# 2

# The International Hospice Movement From the Perspective of the World Health Organization

Jan Stjernsward, M. D., Ph.D.

We ought to give those who are about to leave life the same care and attention that we give those who enter life: the newborns. Nothing would have greater effect on relieving the pain and suffering of the terminally ill than to implement worldwide the enormous knowledge accumulated by the hospice movement.

I worked for some years in East Africa in an ocean of incurable patients. I realized that in the majority of the world's countries good cancer pain relief and palliative care is the most pragmatic, realistic, and humane goal to accomplish, and something that will have immediate effect. Prevention, early detection, and effective treatment in the early stages of cancer are vital goals that will take much time and effort to achieve. Relief of suffering from terminal cancer is an urgent need that could be the spearhead, the model, for what can be done through a public health approach. When I became Chief of Cancer for the World Health Organization I therefore made palliative care one of the priorities.

## SIZE OF THE PROBLEM

We are all born to die. At present 50 million people die yearly, 39 million in developing and 11 million in developed countries. It is estimated that in 2025 the total number of deaths will exceed 62 million. Currently 9 million people around the world develop cancer. By 2015, this figure is expected to rise to 15 million. Ten million cases, two-thirds of the total, will occur in developing countries where most people with cancer do not even present to medical services.

The size of the population aged 60 years and over is increasing dramatically, and will rise from the present 9. 3% to 15% in the year 2030. Developing countries will see the most rapid increase in proportion of elderly people. This proportion will double in 40 years. There will be an even greater need for palliative care in the future, but it will have to be provided by a proportionately decreased working age population of caregivers, equal to tax payers.

## EXAMPLES OF SITUATIONS IN DEVELOPING COUNTRIES

The great majority of new cancer patients, elderly and dying, are in developing countries. Most cancer patients in these countries are incurable, if ever diagnosed at all. For cancer control, these countries have only 5% of the global resources, as compared to 95% for the smaller number of patients in the developed countries.

In Black Africa there are fewer than 100 full-time cancer specialists of any kind for 300 million people. In Indonesia, 33,000 cancer patients are seen every year out of an estimated 240,000 cases. In India there are ten comprehensive cancer treatment centers providing full oncology services, but they cover only 10% of the population. Bangladesh, with 120 million people, has only one cobalt therapy unit, and it dates from 1965, with the cobalt source having remained unchanged over the ensuing three decades. In spite of this limitation, the Bangladesh unit made it a priority to register cancer and start surveillance studies. They mobilized outside support and used the $2 million raised for this purpose. This was a dubious priority for utilization of the funds, especially since the cancer incidence could already have been extrapolated from 40 years of population base registries in India. It can also be considered unethical to diagnose cancer without offering either meaningful therapy or palliative care. There are still 51 countries where there is no legal available morphine or weak opioids.

Many developing countries still have a strong, supportive three-generation family network. The most realistic approach for achieving a meaningful coverage of palliative care would be to empower the family. In developing countries, the future of effective palliative care is less medical than socioeconomic, ethical, and managerial. Preserving and supporting valuable cultural attitudes toward elderly persons and the meaning of dying and death would have far greater impact than purely technomedical advances for years to come.

## WHAT TO DO

The enormous knowledge achieved in cancer palliative care over the past decades from hospices should be implemented in a rational way, with the goal being to benefit as many terminally ill people as possible. It should also include care at the end of the life of elderly persons, individuals with symptomatic chronic diseases, and AIDS patients.

## POLICIES

Globally, palliative care is a neglected area. The need today is enormous and will increase dramatically in the near future. The size of the problem must be made clear to both individuals and society, especially policy makers and the medical profession. They must recognize that something really can be done. They must know that relatively inexpensive, effective, and scientifically valid methods exist for palliative care. It is tragic to see how almost all efforts and resources in the developing countries go to therapeutic approaches, with indeed very limited effect. A striking fact often seen in these countries is the almost complete lack of effort and resources for palliative care. For years to come, before a search for early referral and the training of enough therapists has borne fruit, palliative care will be the only pragmatic and humane solution.

With limited resources worldwide for palliative care, rational approaches are indispensable. Even limited resources stand a chance of making an impact, provided that the relevant priorities are set and effective strategies implemented. Palliative care should attract more of the available cancer control resources in both developed and developing countries. It should be an integral part of cancer care from the very beginning. Curative and palliative care are not mutually exclusive. Palliative care should be an alternative at the time of diagnosis and not seen as a "wastebasket" alternative. Ideally, a person from palliative care should be included upfront in the multidisciplinary team from the first time the patient is seen.

## COVERAGE

A principle of public health approaches has been that a search must be made for scientifically valid methods that are acceptable and maintainable on the community level. This is exemplified by the consensus established by WHO in 1982, with international experts, that (1) drugs are the mainstay of cancer pain relief and (2) a relatively inexpensive, easily applicable approach exists. Known as the three-step pain ladder, this approach has become accepted worldwide and, following a period of field testing, is now being implemented in more than 60 countries.

Taking into account the available resources, it is certain that the principles of the above approach must be followed to achieve coverage—and not only the old conventional institutionalized approach. However, centers of excellence are needed, and as such they must also include training and education.

Governments and professional organizations should ensure that the relief of cancer pain and palliative care programs are incorporated into existing health care systems; separate systems of care are neither necessary nor desirable.

In advocating "Why not freedom from cancer pain?", WHO recommends that countries first establish three specific measures:

• Governmental policy
• Education
• Drug availability

These are the foundation measures. They cost very little, but can have large effects. However, their establishment requires persons with vision, commitment, and leadership. All three areas must be established. Achieving two areas without the third will severely limit the effect. For example, the establishment of a national policy on relieving cancer pain and success in educating the public, healthcare professionals, and policymakers will be inadequate if the necessary drugs (especially the opioid analgesics) are not available for the patients.

During the past several years, there has been growing evidence that national governments are beginning to recognize and to declare the importance of pain relief and terminal care as part of their countries' health priorities. In addition, palliative care and/or pain relief have also been declared as part of the establishment and implementation of national cancer control policies and programs. Among the many countries that have or are planning to establish national palliative care programs, either separately or as part of their national cancer control programs, are Argentina, Cameron, Colombia, Chile, Cuba, Greece, Indonesia, Jordan, Lebanon, Malaysia, Morocco, Oman, South Africa, and Zimbabwe.

Fortunately, there are many examples of progressive steps to cancer pain relief worldwide. Malaysia has changed its laws so that morphine can be made available. This is a great step forward in a country where there is capital punishment for drug peddling. Palliative care is part of their national cancer control program, and there are today five very active and progressive hospice/palliative care centers in Malaysia. Zimbabwe has the "island hospice" that now also is providing coverage by a full-time nurse, thereby empowering the six provincial hospitals. The country is producing its own oral morphine tablets as part of its national cancer control program. India made cancer pain relief a priority in its national cancer control plan in 1986. The three southern Indian states have introduced their own policies.

The pioneering efforts of the Wisconsin Pain Initiative, which also serves as a WHO demonstration project, has lead the way in the United States, where more than 40 states have now adopted their own pain initiatives.

The province of Catalonia, Spain has succeeded in extending palliative care to over 40% of its terminal cases in a short time through establishing clear policies and rational approaches. They created 51 palliative care teams. These include 34 community and 8 hospital teams, in addition to 9 referral units. The goal of the visionary Catalonian leadership is to extend such care to at least 80% of the population of 6 million within the next 5 years in a multidisease approach that encompasses not only cancer patients but also the elderly terminally ill and AIDS patients. Using morphine for pain relief as an indicator for evaluation, they have found that total consumption in the first 3 years increased from less than one kilogram to over 36 kilograms. The province of Las Palmas has already achieved its goal of enabling 80% of their terminally ill patients to die where they choose. In their population of 350,000 people, morphine consumption increased from 37 grams to 4 kilograms. Las Palmas has effective coverage by home care teams. Moreover, the economic savings were considerable. Hospital costs decreased and hospital beds became available for other patients.

The WHO demonstration projects in Wisconsin, Catalonia, and Las Palmas have shown that meaningful coverage and effective pain relief can be achieved with the right leadership, for reasonable costs, and within a relatively short time period.

## DRUG AVAILABILITY

WHO has published guidelines for opioid availability. Some drugs, especially oral morphine, are essential for effective control of moderate to severe pain in most patients. The International Narcotics Control Board (INCB) has also called on governments to reevaluate their needs for opioids in the treatment of pain, especially cancer pain.

Over the past few years, there has been increasing evidence that once vague and ambiguous laws and regulations at state and national levels are being revised to accommodate the legitimate use of opioids, especially for patients with chronic, intractable pain. Methods of assessing and monitoring the medical need for opioids are being improved. These changes are reflected in the substantial increases in the estimated annual requirements for morphine in various countries, as reported to the INCB.

Morphine consumption has increased rapidly since the inception of the WHO cancer pain relief program in 1984. Global medical morphine consumption was relatively constant, at about two tons, between 1972 and 1984. Consumption then started to increase and by 1992 was 10 tons. Today, morphine consumption is estimated to be 12 tons, with a projected rise to 25 tons annually within the next two decades. However, most morphine use in the world continues to be localized in ten industrialized countries that have consistently ranked highest: Australia, Canada, Denmark, Iceland, Ireland, New Zealand, Norway, Sweden, the United Kingdom, and the United States.

In 1993, approximately 120 countries, representing more than 80% of the world's population, consumed only 23% of the total morphine used in the world. These are mainly but not exclusively developing countries in Asia, all of South America, Africa, Eastern Europe, and the Mediterranean region. There may be small quantities of opioids in some hospitals in these countries, but most cancer patients have extremely limited access to opioids, if at all. There are still about 50 countries with no oral morphine available. In these countries, most cancer patients are also incurable, and symptom control is at present the only pragmatic and realistic approach that could be offered.

WHO has advocated the establishment of clear palliative care policies, including opioid availability, over the years. A rational approach to speed up the implementation of adequate pain programs could begin with regional meetings that bring together national drug regulators, pharmacists, palliative care doctors and nurses, and representatives from the drug industry. Such a regional workshop was held recently in Florianapolis, with recommendation made for opioid availability in Latin America. These recommendations were established following a careful situation analysis and identification of impediments to achieving the goal. This successful workshop could serve as a good example for other regions of the world.

## EDUCATION

WHO helped to develop the first international consensus that drugs are the mainstay of cancer pain relief, and then established the three-step pain ladder, allowing public health dissemination of the knowledge gained by the hospice movement. These initiatives have been followed by the establishment of policies for implementing existing knowledge and continuing the educational efforts. A second updated version of *Cancer Pain Relief* has been produced (1995), together with *Guidelines for Opioid Availability, Symptom Relief in Terminal Illness*, and *National Cancer Control Programs: Policies and Managerial Guidelines*. The International Association for the Study of Pain has contributed to this effort with the publication of *Cancer Pain Relief and Palliative Care in Children.* (in press).

A *Manual for Homecare Givers* is now under production to help developing countries achieve coverage. The Phillipines have already produced their own culture-specific version. The quarterly journal *Cancer Pain Release* is an important tool in the international communication effort. WHO collaborating centers, demonstration projects, and focal points around the world are crucial for carrying out the mission.

In many developing countries, the implementation must be carried out one step it to time, as there is no critical mass of professionals to advocate from the beginning. Therefore we recommend the stepwise approach, starting with a centrally located, high-level center.

Continued advocacy for palliative care is important, with particular attention to the public health and pragmatic approach for developing countries. Numerous international workshops and large congresses are being addressed, as is the health profession in editorials and the general public through press releases. Several informative and emotionally engaging films exist that ought to be shown more often on public television.

## CONCLUSION

Over the years, leaders in the field have demonstrated that major symptoms can be controlled and efficient terminal care can be given. Large organizations such as the World Health Organization have produced state-of-the-art consensus reports together with practical guidelines that have been field-tested, as well as policies on how best to implement knowledge gained in palliative care. Numerous national policies are becoming established, directives for professional education in palliative care are emerging, and vital drugs are becoming available. Excellent journals and associations and regular forums for palliative care have been created over the past few years, stimulating a rapid change of information and ideas.

Nothing can stop an idea once its time has come. Palliative medicine is here to stay, and will increase in importance over the years. However, if we are to achieve coverage, reaching all those who are in need of palliative care, it is important to remember that compassion is not efficient in relieving suffering unless it is combined with wisdom. It should be a priority to emphasize a public health rather than an institutional, approach.

Ultimately, the most important factor is the individual who makes the difference. Dame Cicely Saunders exemplifies this truth. We now have a worldwide hospice movement full of individuals who are making a difference in their own countries. Many examples of these significant individual activities are given in the present book, activities that are having a strong positive impact on humankind.

# REFERENCES

Bruera, E. et al. (1995). Opioid availability in Latin America: The declaration of Florianopolis. *Support Care Cancer, 3,* 164–167.

Burn, G. L. (1990). A personal initiative to improve palliative care in India. *Journal of Palliative Medicine, 4,* 257–259.

Dahl, J. (1990). The Wisconsin Pain Initiative. *Journal of Psychosocial Oncology, 8,* 225–227.

Gomez-Batista, X. (1994). Catalonia's five year plan: Basic principles. *European Journal of Palliative Care, 1,* 45–49.

Saunders, C. (1979). *The management of terminal disease.* London: Edward Arnold.

Saunders, C. (Ed.) (1990). *Hospice and palliative care: An interdisciplinary approach.* London: Edward Arnold.

Saunders, C., & Baines, M. (1989). *Living with dying: The management of terminal disease* (2nd ed) Oxford: Oxford University Press.

Stjernsward, J. (1985). Cancer pain relief: An important global public health issue. In H. I. Field, R. Dubner, & F. Cervero (eds)., *Advances in pain research and therapy* (vol. 9), (pp. 555–558). New York: Raven Press.

Stjernsward, J. (1988). WHO Cancer Relief Programme. *Cancer Surveys, 7,* 196–208.

Stjernsward, J. (1993). Palliative medicine: A global perspective. In D. Doyle, G. Hanks, & N. MacDonald (Eds)., *Oxford textbook on palliative medicine.* Oxford: Oxford University Press, pp. 807–816.

Stjernsward, J. (1995). Nurses in the front line of palliative care. *International Journal of Palliative Nursing, 1,* 124–125.

Stjernsward, J., & Joranson, D. (1995). Opioid availability and cancer pain: An unnecessary tragedy. *Support Cancer Relief, 3,* 157–158.

Stjernsward, J., Stanley, K., & Tsechkovski, M. (1986) Cancer pain relief: An urgent public health problem in India. *Indian Journal of Pain, 1,* 8–17.

World Health Organization. (1986). *Cancer pain relief.* Geneva: Author.

World Health Organization (1990). *Cancer pain relief and palliative care.* Geneva: Author.

World Health Organization (1995). *Cancer pain relief.* (2nd ed.) Geneva: Author.

World Health Organization (in press). *Symptom relief in the terminally ill.* Geneva: Author.

World Health Organization and International Association for the Study of Pain (in press), *Cancer pain relief and palliative care in children.* Geneva.

# 3

# Worldwide Developments in Hospice Care: Survey Results

**Marilyn Wilson and Robert Kastenbaum**

Every hospice program has its own story to tell. Most of this book is devoted to a sampling of such narratives. There is also value, however, in considering the broader scene. The present status of hospice programs around the world is much different than what could have been observed two decades or even one decade ago. There is little doubt that rapid changes will continue to occur. This chapter offers a limited but useful documentation of the status of hospice programs at the present time. The information provided by 116 programs in 31 nations both extends our knowledge of hospice operations well beyond the Euro-North American orbit, and establishes a baseline for comparing future developments.

The results presented here are limited primarily because we did not ask every question that would be useful to have answered and because we do not have responses from all hospice programs throughout the world. Some hospice programs were unable to provide all the statistical information requested because they lacked the staff time to compile and review records. Perhaps the World

Health Organization will some day undertake a more extensive (and expensive) survey. In the meantime, we feel rather fortunate that so many programs did respond to so many questions. A debt of gratitude is owed to all the hard-pressed hospice directors and staff members who somehow found the time and energy to respond to the questionnaire despite the incessant demands on these resources. We also appreciate the valuable assistance provided by Arizona State University's Department of Communication and, in particular, by administrative assistant Lori Adler.

## DOING THE SURVEY

The survey questionnaire was prepared in consultation with Dame Cicely Saunders and mailed in May and June of 1994 from Arizona State University. A follow-up mailing was sent in January, 1995. A few responses were still being received as late as July, 1995.

## SAMPLE

The sample selected for this survey consists of all hospice or palliative care organizations known to St. Christopher's Hospice Information Service [HIS] at the time of the study, exclusive of England and the United States (each of which is represented by a substantive chapter in this book). The HIS compiles and updates a list of hospice organizations around the world. This list is based on contacts with the organizations. Ever since its inception, St. Christopher's has received numerous requests for information and assistance from people who were attempting to establish or further develop a hospice organization. There have been many repeated contacts with some organizations, while communication with others has been more limited.

There are no firm data on the number of hospice organizations that are operational throughout the world. Furthermore, any number that might be determined at one point of time is likely to be outdated quickly. Some hospices also merge or divide, as well as change structure and function. There are other uncertainties as well. We cannot be sure that all questionnaires reached their addresses, or that all return questionnaires reached us. Mail delivery services in some parts of the world have been impaired by economic and political turmoil and even by violence.

One must exercise caution, then, in generalizing from the present sample. What we have here is a roster of hospice organizations worldwide that have established contact with the "home base," St. Christopher's. There is no way of determining with any degree of confidence how well this sample represents other hospice programs. (Some individual chapters in this book do describe a variety of hospice programs, including programs that were not included in the HIS registry at the time the study was conducted.)

Questionnaires were sent to the 282 hospice programs that were described as operational in the HIS registry. Completed questionnaires were received from 116 programs: a 41.% return rate. (Five other hospice programs sent their regrets at being unable to furnish the requested information at the present time, and several reported that they were not yet operational.)

**TABLE 3.1a Number of Completed Hospice Surveys by Country**

| Country | No. of Surveys |
| --- | --- |
| Argentina | 2 |
| Australia | 18 |
| Belgium | 6 |
| Bermuda | 1 |
| Brazil | 1 |
| Colombia | 3 |
| Finland | 2 |
| France | 17 |
| Germany | 6 |
| Hong Kong | 5 |
| India | 3 |
| Ireland | 1 |
| Israel | 4 |
| Italy | 8 |
| Jamaica | 1 |
| Japan | 1 |
| Kenya | 1 |
| Korea | 2 |
| Malaysia | 2 |
| Netherlands | 1 |
| New Zealand | 5 |
| Nigeria | 1 |
| Poland | 2 |
| Russia | 1 |
| Singapore | 1 |
| South Africa | 4 |
| Spain | 5 |
| Sweden | 3 |
| Switzerland | 5 |
| Taiwan | 2 |
| Zimbabwe | 2 |
| *Total* | 116 |

TABLE 3.1b Number of Completed Surveys by Region

| Region | No. of Surveys |
|---|---|
| Africa | 8 |
| Australasia | 23 |
| Europe | 61 |
| Far East & Southeast Asia | 16 |
| South America | 8 |
| *Total* | 116 |

Completed questionnaires were received from 31 nations: Argentina, Australia, Belgium, Bermuda, Brazil, Colombia, Finland, France, Germany, Hong Kong, India, Ireland, Israel, Italy, Jamaica, Japan, Kenya, Korea, Malaysia, Netherlands, New Zealand, Nigeria, Poland, Russia, South Africa, Spain, Singapore, Sweden, Switzerland, Taiwan, and Zimbabwe. The returns are tallied for countries in Table 3.1a and for world regions in Table 3.1b).

## BASIC FINDINGS

The survey results reported here are those we consider to be of most general interest. A subsequent report will supplement the basic findings with additional information provided by individual hospice programs and with exploration of some of the complexities, variations, and ambiguities involved in attempting to understand such a broad range of programs in so many different countries.

Here we look first at the pattern of hospice establishment worldwide, and then at some characteristics of the people who are being served. Attention then turns to characteristics of the hospice programs, themselves including types of organization, source of funding, staff and volunteer composition, and types of professional and volunteer services offered.

In reading the chapters in this book contributed by individual hospice programs, you will often note the emphasis on rapid change. All reporting hospices had to go through an early developmental process, all have plans for future innovations and expansions, and all must adapt to emergent conditions in their homelands and areas of operation. It is useful to keep in mind, then, the fact that any survey can provide information only on what has already happened and what is happening at the moment. The data made available to us from hospice programs worldwide can be useful as a "snapshot" of current activity and a baseline for comparison with subsequent developments, but not as a once-and-for-all portrait of the dynamic international hospice movement.

## The Growth of Hospice Programs: An International Timeline

The international hospice movement is young. Almost all of the reporting hospice or palliative care programs outside of the United Kingdom and the United States were established from the 1980s to the present. This period of major growth is still in process.

The pervasive nature of this trend can be seen not only in the general world growth of hospice programs (Figure 3.1a), but also in each of the regional patterns (Appendix: Figures 3.1b–3.1f). In Africa, for example, 6 of the 8 hospices were started in the mid-1980s or later. All of the 61 reporting European hospices were started from the early 1980s to the present, and the same holds true for the 16 reporting hospices in the Far East and Southwest Asia. South America is represented by only 8 reporting hospices at present but, interestingly, two of these were established in 1972, among the earliest created after the founding of St. Christopher's and a little ahead of the first modern hospice in the U. S. (New Haven, Conn.).

It is an important historical sidelight that a few hospices did begin their services well before the emergence of the current palliative care movement, and continue to operate today. The existing organizations with the longest record of palliative

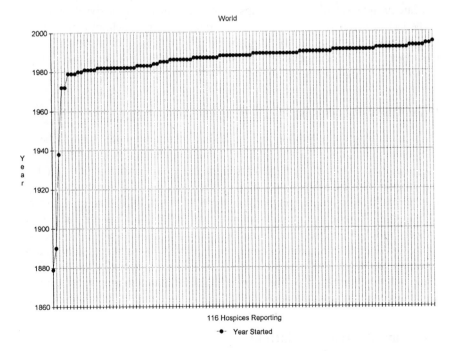

FIGURE 3.1a Year Hospice Started

care service are Our Lady's Hospice (Dublin, 1879); Sacred Heart Hospice (Sydney, 1890); and Caritas Christi Hospice (East Melbourne, 1938). One can go back much further, of course, to (usually) religious organizations that provided comfort to travellers, the homeless, and the poor who would otherwise have been without care and support in their final days (Phipps, 1988; Stoddard, 1978). There have also been some traditional hospitals that earned reputations for their sensitivity to the needs of dying persons, although they would not likely meet the criteria and expectations for hospice programs today.

It may be useful to keep the youthfulness of almost all the reporting hospice programs in mind as we turn to characteristics of the populations served and of the programs themselves. Furthermore, these programs have been and are being established at a particular point in world affairs. Hospice programs that start even a few years from now may find themselves dealing with a significantly different configuration of public and professional attitudes and resource availability, as well as terminal illnesses and their management.

## People Served by Hospice Programs

This section describes several aspects of the population served by hospice/palliative care programs worldwide. Perhaps as important as any of the specific findings is the fact of diversity. There are some marked differences within countries, as well as among countries and world regions. The aggregation of statistical information, then, should not lead us to overlook the characteristics and responsibilities of individual programs.

## How Many People Are Served by Hospice Programs?

There are at least three obvious ways to answer this question: (1) the number of people in the program's cachement area; (2) the number of actual clients; and (3) the proportion of terminally ill patients in the cachement area who are served by the program. We have data on the first and second questions. The third question was not included in the survey because many, if not most, hospices worldwide were not in a position to provide answers. The public health statistical data to answer this kind of question is not available everywhere, and many hospices lack the person and computer resources to compile systematic statistical information, especially beyond the scope of their own daily operations. Several chapters in this book include information on the proportion of the population in need to those actually served in their own areas.

## Cachement Area Populations

Hospice programs were asked to estimate the size (geographical and population) of their cachement areas. There are relationships between geography and population that go beyond what can be presented here. For example, some hospices share the responsibility for the same relatively compact but densely populated urban center, while others are the sole resource for a very large but sparsely populated rural area. It should also be kept in mind that the available data come from a coherent international *sample* of hospice programs, and not from every hospice program in the world.

Taken together, the reporting hospices serve cachement areas with an esti-mated 130 million people worldwide (Figure 3.2a; please see Appendix for regional Figures 3.2b–3.2f). Europe (45%) and Far East/Southeast Asia (30%) together count for three-fourths of the total estimated cachement area population worldwide (about 97.5 million). Reporting hospices from South America (10.5%) and Australasia (9.2%) cover cachement areas of approximately 25.6 million. The reporting hospices of Africa have a combined cachement area that is 5.3% of the total sample, representing a little under 7 million.

The great range in size of cachement populations becomes evident when all reporting hospices within a particular world region are presented (Figures 3.2b–3.2f). A marked disparity in size of the cachement populations can be seen among hospices within each of the five regions.

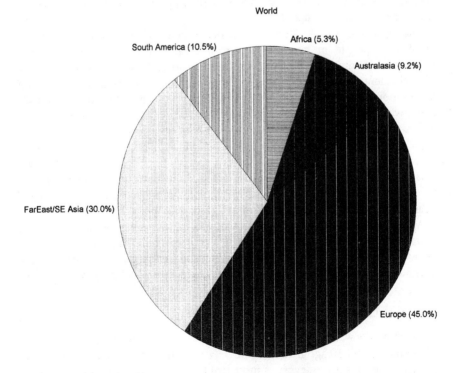

FIGURE 3.2a Estimated Population Served

From these merely statistical findings, one can begin to imagine the differing challenges that are being encountered by the many young hospice programs throughout the world. For example, basic transportation and communication needs are likely to pose major problems in extensive rural areas with difficult access and few telephones. The amount of sheer physical effort and time required to serve a relatively small population in a sprawling area might equal or surpass the person and financial resources needed to serve a large but more compact population in a technologically developed urban area. The sources of stress and concern, as well as the availablity of professional and volunteer caregivers, are likely to differ considerably, even within the same nation or region. In Australasia, for example, one hospice reports a cachement population of about 20 million, while another serves about 50 thousand. We should not be surprised to find differing responses on the part of the hospice organizations, including innovative ways of dealing with distinctive problems.

Of more direct practical value is the number of patients actually seen by hospice programs worldwide (as sampled here). Hospices were asked for the number of clients seen per year. The data supplied were based on either 1993 or 1994, depending on availability. According to their own figures, the reporting hospices served a little under 28,000 patients during the most recent year for which statistics were available.

The regional picture for number of patients served is rather different than the number of people in hospice cachement areas. As we have already seen, Australasia's combined cachement population was but 9.2% of the population for all cachement areas of hospices reporting worldwide. Nevertheless, Australasia served more clients per year (42.4%) than any other region. European hospices, collectively serving the largest percentage of the total world cachement (45%), were second in number of individuals actually enrolled in palliative care programs (31.7%). Hospices in Far East/Southeast Asia served 17.4% of the total clients, followed by South America (4.7%) and Africa (3.9%). It seems remarkable that Asia has moved so rapidly from lacking hospice programs to now serving nearly 5,000 people a year within this survey sample alone, and comprising such a substantial proportion of the total sample (Figure 3.3a).

Again, inspection of individual hospices within each region reveals substantial differences in number of clients served per year (Appendix: Figures 3.3b–3.3f). It seems reasonable to expect that the number of clients served per year will increase most rapidly for the hospices that are in the earliest phases of their development.

## Age and Gender of Patients

Throughout the world and in every region, the largest number of hospice patients fall within the 60–79 age group (Figure 3.4a; Appendix: Figures 3.4b–3-4f). The prevalence of this age category is most strikingly observed in Europe, and least

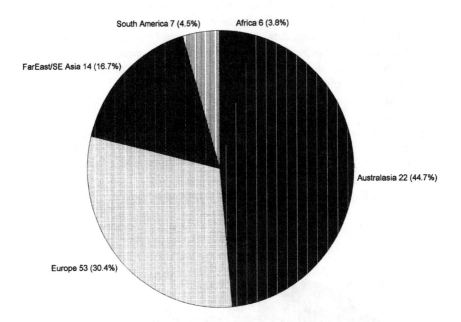

FIGURE 3.3a  # of Clients Served Per Year

apparent in South America. This pattern appears consistent with the global trend toward increased longevity. The oldest age grouping—80+—already contributes nearly 15% of the worldwide hospice case load, a further indication of the role hospice is fulfilling in graying populations.

It is striking, although not unexpected, that only about 11% of hospice patients are under the age of 40 (Figure 3.4a). Accidents, homicide, suicide, and warfare have long taken a high toll among the young, with cancer ranking down the list of major causes of death. It was not uncommon for individual hospices in this sample to report no patients under the age of 19, and some reported none under the age of 39. A more adequate understanding of the age factor would need to include much more information concerning demographic and epidemiological changes on both the macro- and local levels. For example, some areas in various countries have lost many of their younger people to areas that promise better economic opportunities, leaving behind a residual population of older adults with a reduced support system.

Gender differences in utilization of hospice services are not nearly as marked as the age differences already described. Women are in somewhat the majority among patients served throughout the world (Figure 3.5a) . Only in Africa is this difference appreciable, with the female: male ratio approaching 2 : 1. Even here, however, this difference reflects chiefly the all or nearly-all female clientle of two particular hospices (Regional data: Appendix, Figures 3.5b–3.5f). One can find a few other individual hospices throughout the world in which there is a large preponderance of female patients. There are also a few with a male preponderance, although not quite to the same extent.

It would seem that hospice services are being utilized more or less equally by men and women, with some local variations. One might arrive at a different conclusion, however, if these data were examined within the context of changes in longevity and population structure. Women tend to outlive men, with some data indicating that the gender gap in longevity is still increasing. The slightly greater utilization of hospice services by women at present might simply represent the somewhat higher proportion of women in the higher age groupings. Possibly

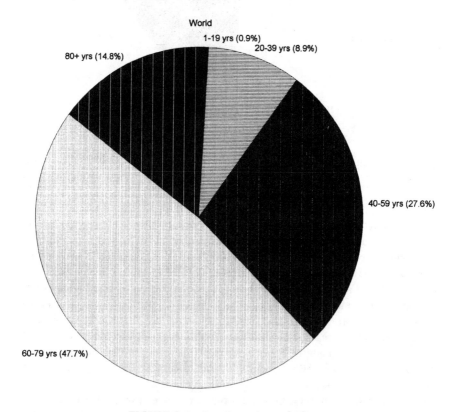

FIGURE 3.4a  Age Groupings of Clients

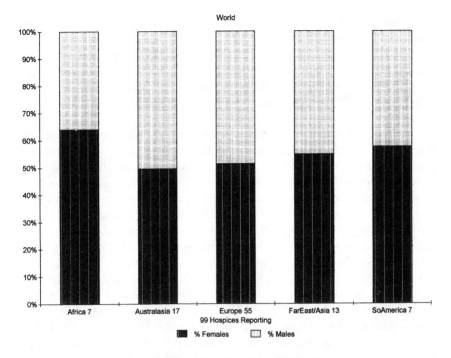

FIGURE 3.5a Ratio of Females to Males

there is *under*utilization by women, taking into account the ratio of elderly women to men who might be in need of palliative care. Investigating this possibility is beyond the scope of the present study.

## Types of Terminal Illness

By far the greatest number of hospice patients had some form of cancer. With one exception, every hospice in the sample reported cancer as the most common condition. The one exception was a hospice in Geneva dedicated to palliative care for people with AIDS (and even here, it is likely that some cancers existed, although considered secondary to the primary cause.)

Hospices differed in the way they recorded, categorized, and reported types of terminal illness. Some hospices indicated that they were unable to keep detailed records because of the pressure of service needs with limited resources. It also seemed that some hospices with case notes available could not afford the staff time required to extract the requested information from their files. The urgent needs of patients and their families rightfully take precedence over recordkeeping and reportmaking. This situation requires us to forego some of the data presentations we had hoped to offer.

There is substantial information, however, on the relative frequency of various types/sites of cancer, as reported by 104 hospices. Worldwise, there was a high incidence group of cancers, respectively, lung, colon, and breast. This was followed by a lower incidence group, respectively, stomach, prostate, cervix, and bladder.

Lung cancer was the most common condition in Australasia, Europe, and Asia. Colon cancer was the most common condition in Africa, and breast cancer most common in Africa and South America. The relatively low incidence of lung cancer in South America (5th among 7 specified cancer conditions) represents one of the most interesting differences among regions. Cervical and prostate cancer had their largest relative impact in South America, coming just behind breast cancer. Bladder cancer was the specified cancer condition with the lowest relative frequency throughout the reporting world hospices, coming at the bottom of the list for all regions exept Africa, where it placed 6th of 7.

It would be useful to know with precision the entire distribution of terminal conditions. Unfortunately, this information cannot be derived with confidence from the survey results. Of the 116 contributing hospices, only 61 (52.6%) provided information on types of terminal illness other than cancer. Often this set of questions was either left blank or was crossed out. Some respondents wrote to the effect that there were so few noncancerous conditions that they did not keep track of them. In this much reduced and, therefore, less representative sample, respiratory disease was the most common noncancer condition reported in Africa, Australasia, and Asia, as well as the second most frequently reported in Europe and South America where, in both regions, infections were cited as the most common. Diabetes was identified as among the most common noncancer conditions only in Asia, where it placed second. Heart disease was reported as the second most common noncancer condition in Africa and Australasia, but down near the bottom of the list in the other regions.

## Characteristics of Hospice Programs

In this section, it is the hospice program itself that becomes the focus. The responding organizations were asked to provide information on the location of their services, sources of funding, staff composition, and services offered by professionals and volunteers.

## Location of Services

Hospice/palliative care organizations may offer their services in various places. Most often, the choices are home, nursing home, hospital, and hospice facility. A given hospice at a particular time in its history might utilize one, several, or all of these alternatives. The reporting hospices indicated as many of these options as they are presently utilizing. In reading Figures 3.6a–3.6f, then, one bears in mind that it is not uncommon for the same hospice to provide its services in more than one location.

Home care is the type of service most often received by hospice clients in every world region (Figure 3.6a: regional data: Appendix, Figures 3.6b–3.6f). As several contributors report in this book, there had been no at-home health care services in their countries or areas until the establishment of the hospice program. It seems clear, then, that hospice programs have already introduced a new dimension to the delivery of health care services in many parts of the world.

The strong emphasis on home care is particularly notable in Africa. In Europe and Asia, there is substantial utilization of all four major options: home, nursing home, hospital, and hospice. Nursing homes do not exist in all hospice cachement areas around the world, however, and sometimes they are not utilized as locations for various reasons. Hospitals are not always readily available to all patients with in a particular cachement area, or may not be receptive to terminally ill cancer patients. Some hospices, then, have a choice of locations for offering

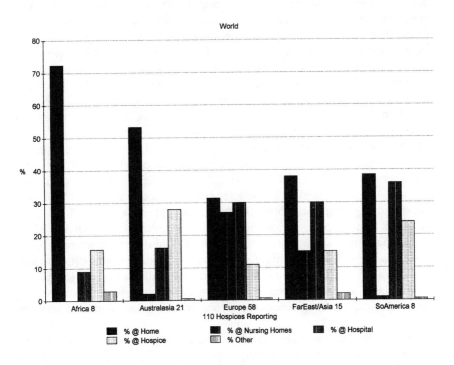

FIGURE 3.6a  Location of Services

their services, and some may have home care (and/or their own inpatient facility) as the only possibility.

Because palliative care at home has been one of the distinguishing features of many early-developing hospice programs, there may have been some inclination to make a virtue out of a necessity. Many of the contributors to this book, however, indicate that hospice directors and caregivers are looking for a balance, in which services can be provided in the location that is most suitable for a particular patient (and family) at a particular point in the terminal process. Perhaps the client's home will continue to be the most common setting for the provision of palliative care; but this picture could change as more hospitals participate more fully in the hospice mission, as more hospices establish their own inpatient facilities, and as innovative alternatives become more available.

## Sources of Funding

There are several ways in which hospice/palliative care organizations can attempt to gain financial support. National and/or local governments might recognize relief of suffering in the terminal phase of life as a legitimate goal of their health care systems and provide funding as a regular budget item. Hospices can also turn for support to private foundations and private individual contributors. In some places, it is possible to apply for special grants to cover hospice expenses, although these seldom if ever pay all the bills or continue over a long period of time. Insurance policies also could help to support hospice care and, with much reluctance on the part of hospice organizations, patients, and their families might be charged fees for the services provided. If this entire spectrum of possibilities falls short in covering hospice expenses—as is almost always the case—the organizations must then turn to a variety of fund-raising endeavors.

Government support now accounts for about half of the funding received by hospices worldwide (as always, within the limits of the present sample). No other source comes close (Figure 3.7a). Individual and regional differences are extreme, however. African hospices as a group, for example, receive less than 7% of their support from governmental coffers (Regional data: Appendix, Figures 3.7b–3.7f). For their own survival, African hospices have had to engage in strenuous fundraising activities which account for about half of their total revenues. Even in regions blessed with relatively substantial governmental support, hospices may still have to divert energies into fundraising. Palliative care organizations in Australasia, for example, receive 63% of their support from the government, but fundraising activities remain the second most effective source of financial aid.

Private contributions from individuals and families provide 9.4% of hospice funding worldwide, but are especially important in Asia, where they account for 23% of the total revenue.

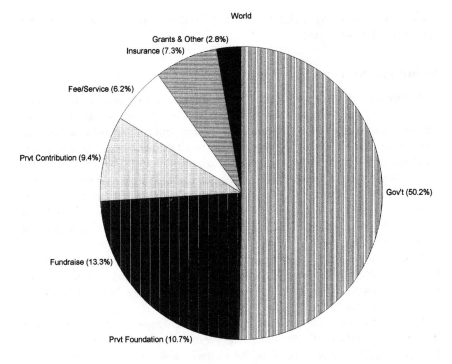

World

Grants & Other (2.8%)
Insurance (7.3%)

Fee/Service (6.2%)

Prvt Contribution (9.4%)

Gov't (50.2%)

Fundraise (13.3%)

Prvt Foundation (10.7%)

FIGURE 3.7a  Sources of Funding

Most, if not all, hospices would prefer to avoid having to charge patients and families for their services, especially people for whom that expense would work a financial hardship. The hospice philosophy includes providing services to all people in need, regardless of their financial situation as well as gender, race, ethnicity, and religion. So far as we can determine, charges are made only in the case of families who are in a position to pay without hardship. It is also likely that the fees for service cover only a portion of the actual expenses involved. No hospice in the sample reported that it had ever turned down a patient because that person could not or would not pay a fee.

Worldwide, about 6% of hospice income derives from fees for service. This figure is seriously skewed, however. In four world regions, fees for service account for less than 5% of the total revenues. In South America, however, fees for service bring in more than a third (34.3%) of the total revenue (Appendix: Figure 3.7f).It will be noted that governmental contributions are slight in this region (6.5%), or about a tenth of the governmental support provided in Australasia and Europe. A hospice-by-hospice analysis would also show that there are often appreciable differences within a region. Some hospices operate within a fairly affluent area, while others serve a population that has lived in economic depression and deprivation for many years.

## Volunteer Services

Community volunteers play a vital role in hospice organizations. House care, personal care, shopping, and transportation are the four most common types of services that volunteers are likely to provide for patients and their families (in addition to indirect services, which include fundraising, accounting, and secretarial functions). Volunteers in many hospices offer all four types of care. Differences in the extent to which various services are offered seem to depend on local conditions. For example, in areas where many clients enter inpatient facilities, there is little need for volunteers to perform personal care. Hospices in different areas of the same country may therefore develop different configurations of volunteer services.

Personal care services are provided by volunteers in all African and almost all reporting European hospices (92.5%). These services also are provided by the majority of Asian (73.3%) and Australasian (61.1%) hospices, but by only 33% of reporting South American hospices.

Transportation services are provided by volunteers most extensively in Australia (94.4 %), Africa (87.5%), and South America (83.3%). The majority of European (72.5%) and Asian (66.7%) hospices also call upon volunteers for transportation services. There are some individual hospices in various parts of the world in which transportation is the only service provided by volunteers.

House care appears to be the most variable or localized of the major services offered by volunteers. It is not unusual for some hospices in the same country to offer, while others do not offer, house care services by volunteers. Furthermore, although none of the reporting African hospice organizations list house care as a regular service provided by volunteers, their accompanying statements indicate that this service, like any others, may be provided if a particular need arises. The special category of "garden care" was noted by hospice service providers in Finland. The short growing season in Finland requires very timely attention if gardens are to prosper; therefore, one of the most heartening services that volunteers can provide is to cultivate and nurture the gardens of terminally ill patients. It is probable that house care is also one of the needs that is most immediately related to the general circumstances of terminally ill patients and their families within the community. Where many client households have dwindled to an elderly person trying to provide care for his or own elderly and terminally ill spouse, there is likely to be more need for house care services than in communities in which large intergenerational households continue to flourish.

The general picture of active volunteer programs does have its gaps. Some of the youngest hospice organizations have yet to establish regular volunteer programs with the appropriate training courses and, particularly in South America, some hospices have only a handful of volunteers.

## Hospice Staffing

Physicians and nurses comprise most of the core personnel of hospice programs worldwide. Some hospices also include social workers, chaplains, specialized therapists (e.g., speech, physical rehabilitation), and pharmacists).

Worldwide, the ratio of nurses to physicians is 4.8:1 (Table 3.2). The ratio of volunteers to nurses is 1:2.3. The ratio of volunteers to total core professional staff (nurses and physicians) 1:1.9.

Regional differences can be seen in hospice staffing patterns (Table 3.2). For example, Africa and Europe differ markedly in the ratio of volunteers to nurses and physicians. Taken collectively, African hospices have a volunteer-to-professional staff member ration that is from two to three times higher than that reported by any other region. European hospices, again taken as a group, actually have a slight preponderance of professional staff as compared with volunteers. Clear differences are also seen in the nurse-to-physician ratio. Australasia's reliance on nurses far exceeds that of South America.

As with all other data reported here, the hospice staff ratios need to be interpreted within the context of national and local practices and circumstances.

What of the other types of service providers? Although medications, especially for relief of pain, are vital to hospice functioning, it is unusual to have a pharmacist on the hospice staff; only 11 were found worldwide in this sample. Social workers, whether full or part-time, are on the staff of 80 (70.1%) of the 114 hospices that reported data on service providers. Australasia differs from the other world regions in that no social workers were reported as hospice staff members. Chaplains are staff members in virtually all African and South American hospices responding to the survey. Worldwide, it is more likely than not to find that a particular hospice program has at least one chaplain who is considered part of the staff. As a number of respondents and chapter contributors have noted, chaplains are usually called upon as the need or patient preference arises, so even hospices without official chaplains do call upon clergy from time to time. Therapists,

**TABLE 3.2 Hospice Staff Ratios**

| Ratios | Africa | Asia | Australasia | Europe | South America | World |
|---|---|---|---|---|---|---|
| Nurses to MDs | 4.2 | 5.1 | 7.1 | 3.9 | 2.6 | 4.8 |
| Volunteers to nurses | 8.1 | 2.9 | 2.7 | 1.2 | 2.7 | 2.3 |
| Volunteers to nurses and MDs | 6.4 | 2.5 | 2.4 | 0.9 | 1.9 | 1.9 |

representing a variety of specialties, are active in hospice programs in every world region, although they are by no means found in every program. There is a tendency for therapists to be part of hospice programs that also include social workers and chaplains, i.e., the larger and more firmly established organizations.

## CONCLUSION

The information supplied by this sample of palliative care programs reveals a young and rapidly developing movement that has been taking hold in all world regions over the past few years. Seeing beyond the numbers, we can sense the energy, excitement, doubts, anxieties, trial-and-error attempts, innovations, disappointments, and achievements that must accompany a pioneering movement that touches on issues of profound human concern. This impression is supported by the following chapters, which describe both the achievements and the continuing struggles of hospice programs throughout the world. It might be well for us to keep in mind that every particular fact about hospice functioning that comes to our attention today is best interpreted within this overall context of new experiences, rapid growth, and all the destabilization involved in the early stages of the creative process.

There is nothing in the present data to indicate that one particular type of hospice configuration is absolutely superior to all others. The variations that can be discerned among regions and among hospices within the same country do not represent negative deviations from a fixed and ideal model, but, rather, a diversity of responses to the diversity of conditions with which palliative care advocates must cope in a particular place at a particular time.

As previously noted, many hospice programs have so many pressing responsibilities that they are limited in the time they can give to keeping and analyzing statistical records of their activities. This problem has the potential for generating "Catch-22" situations, i.e., situations in which one cannot successfully complete Task A without first successfully completing Task B—which, of course, cannot be completed without having first resolved Task A! Hospices will need to document their activities effectively to attract and maintain funding and general public support. The ability to keep learning from hospice experiences also requires statistical documentation, qualitative observations, and the time to reflect on both. One of the emerging challenges for hospice, then, is how to balance the urgent needs of the moment with the long-term needs for collecting and reviewing information. Perhaps the category of "hospice research specialist" should be added to palliative care programs worldwide, with these services contributed on a voluntary basis whenever possible. Research specialists, competent in naturalistic as well as quantitative approaches, might work under the supervision of a coordinator for education and research.

# PART II

# Hospice Experiences Around the World

*Africa*

# 4

# Hospice in Southern Africa

## Peter Buckland*

The Republic of South Africa is situated at the southern tip of the continent of Africa. Geographically, it covers an area roughly the size of continental Western Europe. It has an estimated population of nearly 40 million people, of whom just over 60% live in urban areas. More than 40% of the population are under the age of 16 years and 4% over the age of 65. The other countries of Southern Africa have a much larger rural population than South Africa. To the north of South Africa lies Namibia, Botswana, and Zimbabwe, with Swaziland on its northeast boundary.

## THE EARLY YEARS

The vision and message of hospice was brought to Southern Africa in 1979 by Dame Cicely Saunders. Her visit to the subcontinent was organized by two Cape

* The author acknowledges the source material provided by St. Luke's Hospice (Cape Town), Kath Defilippi (South Coast Hospice), Greta Shoeman (The History of the Highway Hospice), Dave McElvaine (Island Hospice in Zimbabwe) Debra Price (Friends of Swaziland Hospice), and Shelagh Lahoud (Pretoria Sungardens Hospice).

Town medical students, Dr. Christine Dare and Dr. Richard Scheffer. Dame Cicely's visit involved several speaking engagements around South Africa and inspired a number of people to begin the work of gathering like-minded individuals and resources to form the various hospice services in Southern Africa.

In Zimbabwe, Island Hospice was founded in May, 1979; this was probably the first Third World country to start a hospice service. They focused on providing a home care service which they believed would be more cost-effective and would be of greater value to their community than an inpatient unit. (The Zimbabwe experience is reported in detail in Chapter 23.) During 1980, groups began to form in Johannesburg, Cape Town, and Durban, leading to the establishment of hospice services in those cities during 1982 and 1983.

Matron Lyall Cremer founded the Hospice Association of Natal in 1981 to coordinate the development of hospice in that province of South Africa. As in Zimbabwe, most attention was given to the development of a home care nursing team, as there was little or no domiciliary assistance for the terminal patient anywhere in Southern Africa. However, there was also awareness of the need to provide inpatient beds following the model of the British Hospices. In September, 1982, Highway Hospice in Durban admitted the first inpatient, who was cared for in the guest cottage of its founder, Sister Greta Schoeman. In Johannesburg, inpatient's were taken into care during 1985, while St. Luke's Hospice in Cape Town started its inpatient unit in January 1986. Common to all areas, and a pattern which has since been repeated many times over, was the overwhelming support received for the development of hospice from the community itself.

## INVOLVEMENT OF THE MEDICAL PROFESSION

In the early 1980s, the fledgling hospice services throughout the subcontinent were met with skepticism by members of the medical profession. At that time, the service was mostly provided by professional nurses supported by volunteer caregivers. Medical involvement was usually minimal, although much was done to enlist the support of the medical profession and to convince them of the need to prescribe effective pain and symptom control regimes for their patients.

Fortunately, there were some medical practitioners interested in this field of medicine, and they began to provide voluntary medical services to support the nurses working in the field. These doctors primarily educated themselves by reading extensively on the subject. In January 1984, Professor Eric Wilkes from St. Luke's Hospice in Sheffield came to South Africa. His visit played an important role in further influencing medical practitioners of the need to apply the techniques of palliative care. Four years later, Dr. Robert Twycross's visit further enhanced the knowledge of palliative care in Southern Africa.

# PROVIDING THE RESOURCES FOR HOSPICE

Hospice in Southern Africa has grown from a community need to provide support for the terminally ill patient in a home environment. Prior to hospice, patients for whom there was no cure were often left to do the best they could in their home surroundings. Patients fortunate enough to have private medical insurance could afford a private hospital bed and private medical attention to provide some assistance. However, the majority of the South African population did not and still does not have private medical insurance, and therefore, are totally reliant on government medical services for their health care.

Currently, there are 35 hospice services in the Republic of South Africa, two in Botswana, one covering the kingdom of Swaziland, and the Island Hospice Service, which has 16 branches throughout Zimbabwe. There are approximately 15 medical practitioners and 300 professional nurses working in hospice. In addition, there are approximately 3,500 trained volunteer caregivers working alongside the employed professional nurses, medical practitioners, and social workers.

Right from the outset, the philosophy of providing care to the terminally ill patient irrespective of the person's ethnic background, social class, or religion was adopted as the ethos of the hospice movement, and it remains so today. In addition, all hospice services are provided to patients whether or not they can make any financial contribution towards the care they receive. Some of the hospices in South Africa have been able to recover a small proportion of their costs from those patients who have private medical insurance. However, this usually amounts to approximately 10% of the individual hospice's income. Attempts have been made since the early 1980s to influence government to help finance the cost of providing hospice services. Nowhere in the Southern African region has this attempt been successful, and all the hospice services remain financially unsupported by any of the governments in this region.

Therefore, much attention has been given to fundraising programs, as no hospice service can rely on more than 20% of its income being derived from donations made by the patients and their families. Most hospices in Southern Africa run extensive fundraising programs, many of which are conducted entirely by volunteer staff. The larger hospices employ professional fundraising personnel to address this need. Most hospice services in Southern Africa have been success-ful in finding donations to provide the buildings and equipment. However, the difficulty is and always has been the financing of the operational costs of hospices services

## LEARNING AND TEACHING ABOUT HOSPICE

The knowledge and expertise to develop hospice services in Southern Africa was gained through reading books and journals and from sending people to England and the United States for training. In the early years, the hospices closely followed the models of these already established and experienced hospice services. Public relations and education programs were introduced to influence the community and to inform them about what hospice could do to support those caring for a terminally ill patient at home. As a result of these programs, hospice has become an accepted part of the support services for terminally ill patients wherever a hospice service exists in Southern Africa.

Introductory courses are offered to medical and nursing students in all major centers of Southern Africa. Closer involvement has also been established with local state hospitals, oncologists, radiotherapists and chemotherapists. A registered course in basic palliative nursing approved by the South African Nursing Council has recently been introduced by the Hospice Association of Southern Africa, and this is beginning to have an influence on nursing, not only in hospice, but in other health care settings as well.

The Centre for Hospice Learning was founded in 1989 by Hospice Association of Witwatersrand as a National Educational Centre in Johannesburg. Its mission was to facilitate learning about the hospice approach to care and the development of appropriate behavior in the face of death, dying, and bereavement. The Centre for Hospice Learning has played a key role in changing patterns of care for the terminally ill by educating many people about the concept of hospice care.

## DOMICILIARY CARE

Typically, a home care nursing service in Southern Africa consists of at least one or more professional nurses who coordinate the care of the patients at home. They are supported by a medical practitioner, who is most often a general practitioner or a hospital doctor or, in larger hospices, a hospice medical practitioner. In addition, trained volunteer caregivers, together with the family, provide a supportive service to the patient and the professional care team. Every hospice service in the subcontinent provides psychosocial support to the patient and family both during the patient's illness and in the following bereavement period.

## BEREAVEMENT CARE

Most hospices have specially trained bereavement counselors, some of whom hold relevant professional qualifications and who voluntarily provide this service to the immediate family or significant friends. Bereavement or loss counseling has become an important role for hospice in Southern Africa. In the early days of Island Hospice in Zimbabwe, the country had emerged from a bloody struggle for independence, leaving many traumatized families and people. Island Hospice provided a public bereavement service to help address this need and remains a major emphasis in their work. In more recent times, South Coast Hospice in the province of KwaZulu has become involved in providing support for victims of violence, and in training others to provide bereavement and loss counseling.

## INPATIENT CARE

A number of inpatient units have developed in the major centers of South Africa. There are now 11 centers providing just over 100 beds for terminal care. Admission is mostly for pain and symptom management. On average, patients in the inpatient units remain for 10 days, and 40% of admissions are discharged to the care of the home nursing services.

## DAY CARE

Day care is a vital aspect of most urban hospices. In general, day care is provided by volunteers for one or more days each week. With the emphasis on providing "a day out" there is a strong social aspect, together with rehabilitative activities for those who are interested. The character of day care differs from hospice to hospice, as it aims to serve the community in the appropriate manner for that community. One of the difficulties being faced by many hospices is that the concept of a day care center is not always appropriate for the patients. For example, there are centers where driving to attend a day car center could involve spending up to an hour or more in a motor vehicle, which is not always in the best interest of a sick patient.

## VOLUNTEER SUPPORT

Every hospice service in Southern Africa is dependent on volunteer support. Most hospices have a person designated as their volunteer coordinator who organizes regular volunteer training courses, as well as managing and supporting the volunteer groups. The focus of a basic training program is to help the volunteesr come to terms with their own mortality; to understand the philosophy and work of the hospice service; to learn listening skills; to be given basic information about the dying process; and to fulfill the role of a volunteer caregiver in the multidisciplinary team. Some hospices go further and provide counseling training, which requires a much longer preparation and training period.

Experiential learning and role play are regular features of most volunteer training courses, and in most cases self-evaluation and an interview follows completion of the course prior to being accepted as a volunteer caregiver. However, volunteers work in other fields of hospice as well, such as reception, gardening, transport, preparation of meals, administration, and fundraising. Some hospices require compulsory attendance at ongoing training courses as well as attendance at support group meetings. Volunteers involved in caregiving roles are also asked to make regular written reports of their experiences in caring for patients and their families.

## TERMINAL ILLNESS IN SOUTH AFRICA

At first, hospice care in Southern Africa gave most attention to terminal cancer patients. Patients with motor neurone disease, end-stage renal failure, and some other terminal illnesses were also included. During the last few years, the demand for care from patients dying of an AIDS-related illness has become a major concern for the hospice movement. The home care nursing services of the hospices have usually been able to cope with the increased demands made on their services; however, many have had to limit the geographic area which they cover. Inpatient beds, where they exist, have been in regular use by patients requiring pain or symptom relief, family relief, and in some circumstances, during the final days of the patient's life.

Unfortunately, there are no good data available in South Africa about the numbers of people requiring terminal care. However, best estimates seem to indicate that the hospice service is reaching a high percentage of the terminally ill patients within the developed urban areas.

## BUILDING BRIDGES

Hospice in Southern Africa has played an important role in building bridges across racially divided societies. From the outset, hospice has always been a nonracial organization, accepting patients just as they are. However, there has also always been awareness that people of an African culture have different attitudes towards dying than do people of a Western culture. Hospice in Southern Africa, in recognizing this fact, has engaged African staff who understand and are sympathetic to the particular needs of African people.

During the apartheid years there were at times difficulties encountered in providing a home care nursing service to many of the people in urban African townships. These difficulties were caused mainly by the violence within those communities, which made them a so-called "no-go" area at times. Furthermore, many of the urban African people in South Africa live in small homes, often without electricity or running water, and in vastly overcrowded situations compared to Western standards. Hospice over the years has attempted to break through some of the cultural barriers to reach the African people. With the help of the African nurses and trained African volunteers, progress has been achieved in nearly every urban center around Southern Africa.

One example of an urban satellite hospice is in Pretoria. This hospice service started in 1987, and although it drew patients from all communities in Pretoria, it was found that African patients coming to a day care center experienced difficulties with language and cultural barriers. The feeling of the hospice care team was that they were not meeting the needs of these patients or their families, and therefore they decided to open a day care center within the African township itself. They started out by identifying groups of interested people from within the specific African community, particularly doctors working in the area, and others in similar and related organizations involved in those communities. One of the great problems which they encountered was the lack of facilities or services to detect cancer at an early stage. Their experience revealed that when medical help was sought, the disease was already far advanced, and there was rapid progression to the terminal phase. This satellite hospice now has a well-attended day care center run by the local African community.

The model of a satellite hospice operating in an African community usually takes the form of a day care center where patients come together, as well as volunteer caregivers and, frequently, members of the family. They enjoy a day of social activity organized by the volunteers. Nursing and medical attention is available for those patients requiring it, and transport is usually provided where possible. The hospices work also with traditional healers where necessary, as frequently people from African cultures will want to maintain both Western medicine and more traditional treatments for their illness. The challenge facing most hospices in the large urban areas of Southern Africa is finding the resources to expand their services to reach the large numbers of people living in high-density areas, and who live in very poor conditions.

## REACHING RURAL COMMUNITIES

There have also been attempts to reach people living in rural areas. In 1987, South Coast Hospice situated in Port Shepstone on the South Coast of KwaZulu began its rural outreach program. This team worked in conjunction with the Murchison

Mission Hospital to train members of the hospital's nursing and medical teams in the basic aspects of palliative care. They also work with the primary health care nurses employed by the KwaZulu Health Department. These nurses work mostly in the rural communities of KwaZulu, and have undergone the hospice training program, which includes orientation to hospice and a course in basic palliative care emphasizing pain and symptom control. In addition, South Coast Hospice provides a specialist backup service through their inpatient unit in Port Shepstone. These teaching programs and other resources have enabled hospice care to reach many terminally ill people in rural settings.

Similarly, in 1991, hospice in Swaziland commenced through the efforts of a British expatriate, Sister Stephanie Wyer. She inspired the people in Swaziland to join with her to develop Hospice at Home. Today the nurses in Swaziland Hospice at Home cover most of the country, working also in rural areas, and traveling long distances to reach their patients. Some patients have no telephones, so contact is less frequent than would normally be the accepted standard in developed countries. The challenge facing those hospices in Southern Africa who serve large rural communities is to develop mobile hospice services to take hospice to the communities. Often roads are accessible only to four-wheel-drive vehicles, and traveling time can be quite long. Lack of adequate financial resources limits the further development of this aspect of hospice services.

## HOSPICE ASSOCIATION OF SOUTHERN AFRICA

In 1987 the hospices of South Africa joined to form the Hospice Association of Southern Africa. The purpose of this national body was to represent, facilitate, and coordinate development and growth of hospice in the region. Through the auspices of the Hospice Association, a basic caregivers training manual has been written and printed; a six-week course in basic palliative nursing has been developed and implemented; and coordination of national fundraising programs to help support the work of all hospices is underway, as well as the development of national information and promotion campaigns.

## RECENT DEVELOPMENTS

One aspect of hospice in Southern Africa which has come to the fore in the last six or seven years has been the need to move away from the Western models. Innovative ideas are needed to reach people in rural communities as well as serve people in high-density, poverty-stricken urban communities. Furthermore, the pandemic of AIDS is a major concern of all hospice services in this region.

Most hospice services recognize that they cannot possibly cope with the number of projected terminal patients affected by the AIDS pandemic. Therefore, emphasis is now being placed on increasing the training and education programs to mobilize more people in the community, as well as other community services, to help share responsibility for caring for more terminally ill people in the future. The constraint of having to generate all their own funding in order to provide the best services possible is a heavy burden for all hospice services.

The home care nurse in Southern Africa has greater challenges than most, as she is often the only professional resource available to a family caring for a terminal patient. Legislation in Southern Africa prohibits nurses from prescribing medicines, and they often have to rely on persuasion and personal influence to obtain a prescription from medical practitioners who know little or nothing about palliative care regimes.

There are encouraging signs that more and more communities are prepared to take responsibility for providing hospice services within their community. It is hoped that this continued growth and involvement will help hospice in this region to eventually persuade the governments in the various countries to take a stronger and more positive interest in palliative care, and to recognize its importance as part of the wider health care service in their country.

## RESEARCH

Little research has been conducted in Southern Africa, owing to financial constraints and the time pressure experienced by the people working in hospice. Perhaps in the future and with new funding we might be able to achieve this objective.

## CONCLUSION

The success of hospice in Southern Africa has been the substantial voluntary contribution of many thousands of people over the past 15 years. Many people have contributed thousands of rands and dollars, mostly without recognition, in order to fund this service. Hospice in Southern Africa is a living memorial to the many courageous people who have been cared for, and to the many who have contributed much and asked nothing. One of our dreams is to establish a Chair of Palliative Medicine in one or more of the university medical faculties. Hospice in Southern Africa continues to endeavor to secure government funding for this region and to have hospice recognized as an important component of the health care system. Hospice's involvement is essential to the development of primary health care services in this region.

Hospice Southern Africa's message to people in other developing countries around the world is not to be daunted by the challenges of providing hospice care.

- *Start small, involve a few people who share the vision, and commitment, and begin to work to bring about the change.* Hospice is "infectious," and other people in the community will soon rally around to support it.
- *Don't rely on government support or assistance,* because the priorities in developing countries are usually far more focused on keeping people alive than on helping to care for them through the last stages of a terminal illness.
- *Look to other developing countries for your model of care* and not to the developed countries of Western Europe and North America. Developing countries don't have the resources, either financial or human, to match the services provided in the developed countries, nor is the range of medicines available in those countries always available in developing countries.

While hospice is very definitely about relief from pain and other distressing symptoms, let us also not forget that hospice is all about people caring for people.

# 5

# Zimbabwe: The Island Hospice Experience

## D. McElvaine

The story of Island Hospice Service started in 1977 with the diagnosis of cancer in a 20-year-old university student, Frances Butterfield. Her illness and subsequent death in November of that year led her parents to evaluate the level of care and support that they and their daughter had received prior to her death. They also examined in a critical, yet very personal, manner how they were dealt with as bereaved parents after their daughter's death.

This family's intensely painful experience resulted in the realization that a service was needed to assist other people who faced similar situations. They envisaged a service, rather than a place. This service would address the physical, emotional, and spiritual needs of those with a life-limiting illness; their families; and bereaved people. At that time, the hospice movement was gaining momentum in the United Kingdom and the United States. Frances' mother travelled to St. Christopher's Hospice in London for a closer look at the services and facilities offered.

She returned to Zimbabwe convinced that our community did have a need for some type of hospice service. A few days after her arrival, she had the opportunity of travelling to Pretoria in South Africa to meet Dame Cicely Saunders—a woman whose sense of purpose and compassion was comparable to her own. She then consulted a lecturer in psychology at the local university to ascertain the next step.

They decided to hold a public meeting at the university to assess the level of interest and concern.

Their initial trepidation proved to be unfounded—this meeting in May, 1979 was filled to overflowing with people from all walks of life, many of whom had undergone similar experiences. A questionnaire was given to each person. The vast majority indicated that they would be prepared to support and work with any formal organization which resulted.

A constitution was drawn up, and Island Hospice service was established and registered in the first month. It had become the first hospice in Africa.

In addition, Zimbabwe was the first Third World country to start its independent career (in April, 1980) with an active hospice program already in operation. The name was taken from the writings of English poet and cleric John Donne (1975, p. 103):

> No man is an island, entire of itself. Every man is a part of the continent, a piece of the main, and each man's death diminishes me because I am involved in mankind.

During the first year after registration, numerous group meetings and discussions were held in private homes. This broad self-educative experience provided what was then a fledgling organization with a sound base of knowledge and skill on which to build further activities. Those in the helping professions, such as medicine, nursing, psychology and social work, were actively recruited. Their academic and professional input was of great value, along with the contributions of those who had experienced illness and bereavement.

Many doctors at the time regarded Island Hospice with a degree of skepticism and distrust. On one occasion, for example, our pioneers were described by a specialist physician as "a group of middle-aged nursing sisters and matrons who have nothing better to do with their time." An even less complimentary description came from another doctor who characterized our volunteers as "the death-watch beetles." The people who made this type of observation may have felt threatened by a move to demystify medicine and question their knowledge base and practices. Until then, the focus of medicine had been primarily physiological, in contrast to the holistic approach taken by hospice, which considers all aspects of a person's illness.

There were, however, a large number of professional people who had recognized a real gap in our health services through their own practices. These professionals were also prepared to increase their own knowledge. Until last year, our various chairpersons deliberately were drawn from the medical field. An eminent physician was appointed as medical director. These moves did much to allay the fears and suspicions of his colleagues.

Zimbabwe's pre-independence history also had a marked effect on public opinion regarding death and bereavement. The bloody and protracted struggle for independence had personally affected hundreds of thousands of people. The need for skilled bereavement care was at its zenith when Island Hospice was formed. These large-scale events, coupled with our early focus on public relations and education, were strong contributory factors to our successful establishment and have remained crucial to our continued functioning.

In line with our principles of continuing education were our contacts with other hospice groups. In 1980, our medical director toured several United Kingdom hospices. Soon thereafter two of our voluntary nurses went on an intensive placement, again in UK hospices. This policy of continuing education is ongoing, as finances permit, but applies only to courses and conferences that are of direct professional benefit to our work, rather than "conference attending" merely for public relations and networking purposes. In addition, we have actively assisted with the establishment of other hospices, both in Zimbabwe and in the Southern African region.

A major feature which contributed to our early establishment and, indeed, our current functioning, has been our financial accountability. Our first treasurer was the managing director of an international trust and investment company. All subsequent treasurers have been very prominent figures in the financial market. These appointments have contributed to the public's belief—which is entirely accurate—that our finances are carefully husbanded and meticulously dispersed. Many of our links with the business community have been forged through personal and professional acquaintances with leaders in commerce.

## ISLAND HOSPICE SERVICE TODAY

Our current practices are carefully designed to continue justifying this support. Our financial dealings are completely transparent, and it is a measure of our achievements that our running costs, which are currently in excess of Z$2,000,000 each year, are met primarily by local resources and donations. It is only in recent years that international donor funding has been sought for specific development projects. All donors to date have professed themselves well pleased with the way in which their contributions have been utilized.

In our early days, we were fortunate to secure the services of several volunteer professional people whose spouses were financially supportive of their work with Island Hospice. Fundraising has always been a major component of our activities, and in recent years we have engaged a fundraiser/public relations officer on normal terms of employment to coordinate our activities in this field. This is an innovative step in a Third World country. We have seen a move away from relying entirely on "special events" fundraising to income-generating projects. We now run numerous projects, such as the sale of donated secondhand articles and clothes; a magazine exchange system; collection boxes in hundreds of retail outlets; and the like. We have very close links with service clubs such as the Lions, Rotary, and Round Table. At present, we also have financially advantageous contracts with all medical insurance firms.

In general, we are regarded as a "popular" organization by the public, from large commercial concerns down to nursery school children. Apart from our educational achievements, this perception is itself contributing significantly to our continued financial viability.

As indicated, Island Hospice started with a group of volunteer workers, but we have since found it necessary to employ salaried staff as the organization has grown. In Harare, we currently employ over 30 staff members, 70% of whom are professional nurses and social workers. Our volunteer network has also grown concurrently, enabling us to continue providing a full and free community service.

We have several categories of volunteers:

1. *General members* who pay an annual subscription, receive our newsletter, but are not actively involved in our work.

2. *Those who have attended an induction course* so that they can make an informed decision as to the type and extent of their involvement with us. After this course, some people become involved in administration and fundraising, while others state a preference for future direct patient/client contact.

3. *Those who are given duties on a roster basis* to assist in reception for a period of approximately 6 months. They do not carry a caseload during this time, but invariably have some contact with patients, their families, and bereaved people. These experiences give them the opportunity to decide whether they would like to continue their involvement in direct care. In addition, their performance is closely monitored. Prior to our 2-week training course, potential caregivers are asked to provide references and undergo a formal interview. The training course has an extensive theoretical base at a layperson's level, and includes many roleplaying exercises. These exercises enable our staff to evaluate the participants. The course concludes with a second formal interview during which strengths and weaknesses are explored, together with an examination of individual future development. Within 2 months, those caregivers who have "passed" the foregoing attend a 1-week bereavement course. If they are still found to be suitable, they are assigned to actively assist our professional staff under the close supervision of our caregiver coordinator.

At the beginning, the demand for our service came mostly from bereaved people. No other organizations were offering bereavement support at that time. Our bereavement service continues to be available to families whether or not the deceased had been in our care. However, the demand for patient care increased rapidly as more medical practitioners realized that we could offer a specialized palliative care service. This demand has been exacerbated by the AIDS pandemic. More than 90% of our patients have cancer, but an increasing number of these cancers are AIDS-related.

Given this trend and its economic implications for further expansion of our staff, we have decided to expand and formalize our external training facilities. We have always given talks to both interested groups and professional people, such as post-basic nurses and medical students. Increasingly we now see our role as being more specialized and training-oriented.

We believe that in the 16 years since our establishment, Island Hospice Service has accumulated a high degree of knowledge and practical expertise. We wish to empower other community groups to take both patient and bereavement referrals and give adequate care. In the past, our training of such groups was somewhat sporadic and reactive. Now, however, thanks to donor funding, we employ a training officer whose role it is to develop proactive training at all levels in the community.

We are firmly of the opinion that palliative care needs to be part of the mainstream health service, and were instrumental in securing funding for the establishment of a National Palliative Care Coordination post in the Ministry of Health last year. We also aided in the selection of a suitable director, and since her appointment have worked closely in the program of regional palliative care workshops for doctors and nurses employed by the Ministry of Health. Our medical student training program has been extensively reviewed and increased, as has our education input to other groups.

With this structure now firmly in place, we anticipate that an ever greater proportion of our population will have access to decent palliative care at all levels of the health system. Concurrently, we are also critically evaluating the extent of our involvement with "outside" bereavement referrals, which currently comprise approximately 40% of the workload of our social work department.

From the start, our intention was to offer home care, as opposed to an inpatient facility. There were two reasons for this decision. The first was the obligation to make the most effective use of our scarce resources. Home care seemed to be the most viable option, given the very high cost of inpatient units and the desire of most people to die in a home setting. Secondly, our approach has always been holistic. The focus has always been on the patient and family as a unit, rather than the patient in isolation. Subsequent bereavement counselling is generally enhanced if the counsellors have been involved with the whole family prior to death.

## WORK IN PROGRESS

In the back of our minds, however, there always was the hope that one day we would be able to open our own inpatient unit. To date, this has not been achieved. Given our emphasis on increased training and the incorporation of palliative care into the whole health system, we are now exploring the possibility of establishing such a unit in an existing ward of Harare's major teaching hospital. We envisage that such a unit would be staffed by government-paid nurses who would work under our direction. As a further extension of this plan, we hope to establish a hospital advisory team and are currently seeking funding to employ a medical officer. The doctors who presently assist Island Hospice do so on a voluntary basis, and their time is thus rather limited. Several charitable organizations in Zimbabwe have managed to secure government funding for a proportion of their staff salaries, and we had always hoped that Island Hospice would be able to tap into these resources. Efforts to date have been unsuccessful, however, and the current economic standing of the government makes it highly unlikely that we will receive financial assistance from this source.

Although our plans for an inpatient unit were somewhat vague, another, more clearly envisaged goal has been realized. A specific gift made it possible to establish a day care center in February, 1992. What we did not envisage, however, was that we would be forced to close this facility 3 years later. It was being underutilized by the majority of our patients and was tying up valuable staff and office space resources. In retrospect, it was evident that a more thorough needs assessment of this facility should have been conducted prior to its establishment.

In sharp contrast, a development that we had never envisaged has proven to be extremely valuable. A donation by a motor corporation provided us with a fully equipped ambulance. We subsequently leased this vehicle to a medical emergency response company with the proviso that, in addition to meeting all related costs, this company will make the vehicle and its crew available to us free of charge whenever we require it for a patient in our care.

In retrospect, there are several areas of our operations which should have been more closely examined and dealt with some time ago. One of these areas is accomodation. Currently, we lease a large section of a building that belongs to and is partially occupied by the Cancer Association. The rental we pay for these facilities is minimal, but we are currently faced with a shortage of office space. The Cancer Association itself is expanding. This situation has led to the physical fragmentation of our departments. We should have recognized some time ago that our inevitable expansion eventually would require us to have the security of our own premises.

Another current problem area is one that should have been addressed at our formation in 1979. There are currently 17 branches of Island Hospice Service throughout Zimbabwe. Four of these branches utilize paid staff as well as a volunteer network. Our founders were understandably keen to assist with the establishment of other branches. Insufficient attention was paid, however, to the organizational and financial implications of having branches which used our name and welfare organization number.

In practical terms, each of our branches conduct their own affairs and are financially autonomous. Legally, however, Island Hospice Service, Harare, could be liable for their assets and liabilities. Paradoxically, we have neither the facilities nor even the mandate to monitor their activities. We are currently negotiating to have each branch registered as a separate welfare organization. Once this is achieved, we would form a National Council whose role it would be to monitor and register/deregister branches. The National Council would also engage in national fundraising and training programs. A major role of such a body would be the establishment of standards of care which could then be enforced to provide a uniformity of service to the whole of Zimbabwe.

Without any doubt, we feel that our most significant accomplishment over the years has been the increase in "home deaths" and the concurrent change in the attitudes of both the general public and human service professionals (particularly doctors) to death and bereavement. When we first started keeping proper statistics in 1981, only 14% of our patients died at home. Last year this figure had risen to nearly 80%.

We believe there is an increasing openness to speaking of and dealing with the previously taboo subjects of illness and death at all levels and ages of our multicultural society. A very substantial proportion of our funding comes from the 25–50-year-old age group, including those who have not looked after a family member. Our popularity in the community is a source of great satisfaction and a sense of achievement.

Some of our plans for the future have already been covered, e.g., in-patient unit, employed doctor, hospital advisory team, reregistration of branches. However, there are also management issues to which further attention needs to be paid. One of these issues is concerned with the role of our Board/Executive Committee. Our first Committee members were all service professionals in their own right. It was largely due to their knowledge and dedication that Island Hospice developed in scope and professionalism. However, as the organization grew, their input was needed less on professional issues and more on service delivery and long-term financial planning. As such, a more business-oriented approach is needed. We believe that our Executive Committee now should consist primarily of successful business people who will encourage and allow paid management to administer the day-to-day functioning of Island Hospice.

I am very conscious of the fact that this report contains no academic reference material. Although we have a great deal of clinical knowledge and experience—and have been described as "the mother of hospice in Africa"—our contribution to international conferences, journals, and the like has been woefully inadequate.

Financial and time constraints to date have simply not allowed us to be active on the international scene, but it is hoped that the present publication will stimulate such a move. Whilst we are totally against "conference-trotting," we do need to pay further attention to networking and establishing our international credentials if our plans to be further regarded as an educational facility are to be successful.

With regard to our own practices, I believe that a valuable area of research could be centered around the public perception of our activities. Research would also be useful with regard to characterizing certain kinds of death as being either "good" or "bad." Our judgment does not always accord with the family's recollection and perception of a death. When people work in a highly emotional human service field, it is easy to point to the fulsome praise received in verbal and financial terms as meaning that we do no wrong. This assumption might prevent us from recognizing how our practices could have been improved. I believe that we would do well to become more objective about the delivery of palliative and bereavement care as professional services.

To those who are considering the establishment of a hospice or palliative care program, our advice would be to start small but think big. Before moving into an area of service, we recommend a very careful prior examination of existing resources. This process will enable you to include, rather than oppose, existing programs, thereby preventing duplication and overlap. Education and public relations are essential parts of any palliative program, particularly if the resources come from the community. The program must be perceived as benefitting the entire community, rather than a select group. Our experiences have shown us that home care is the most viable broad-based option in terms of holistic care and the utilization of limited resources.

Above all, we would counsel that the client's needs and those of his/her family always be considered paramount. The hospice movement arose partly in reaction to depersonalized medical care. If we lose our humanity and our listening skills, we will lose the essence of a thoroughly caring program.

## REFERENCE

Donne, J. (1971, Original 1628). *Devotion*. Ann Arbar: University of Michigan Press.

# The Americas

# 6

# Bermuda: The Patients Assistance League and Service (P.A.L.S.)*

## Ann Smith Gordon, R. N. J. P.

## BACKGROUND

P.A.L.S. is a registered Bermuda charity dedicated to providing cancer patients with quality care, primarily in the home setting, and at no charge, regardless of their financial circumstances. A few words about Bermuda will be useful in setting the context for the development and activities of P.A.L.S.

These beautiful islands lie very much alone in the vast North Atlantic Ocean at 32 degrees latitude. The nearest landfall is North Carolina, 600 miles to the West, while New York is some 700 miles away. Bermuda is still occasionally confused with the far away Bahamas and West Indian Islands found 1,000 miles to the South.

* Our most sincere gratitude to The Bermuda TB, Cancer and Health Association, which has kindly provided P.A.L.S. with office and storage space at their premises for many years; The government of Bermuda for recognition and support of our work: The Executive Committee and long-serving volunteers of P.A.L.S.; to all those hundreds of local and international businesses, banks, clubs, schools, individuals, and charitable organizations who support P.A.L.S. financially and in so many other imaginative and special ways; and particularly to Mrs. Hilary Soares, R.N., whose recognition of the need of a home care service for cancer patients led her to create P.A.L.S.

The remote Bermuda Islands, 21 square miles in area, are linked today to the rest of the world by jet aircraft and ships of all descriptions, but were uninhabited until a British sailing ship called "the *Sea Venture*" was wrecked on its protective but treacherous reefs in 1609. Colonized by the British in 1612, life was extremely difficult through the ages, though today Bermuda enjoys one of the highest standards of living in the world, and its 60,000 people are among the most charitable to be found anywhere.

Hospice and palliative care as we understand it today was relatively unknown, and certainly an untried and unpopular subject in Bermuda, until 1979, when a physician from the Royal Victoria Palliative Care Unit in Montreal, Canada came to Bermuda to speak to local physicians on the subject of pain control in palliative care. In the same year Mrs. Hilary Soares, R.N., was appointed oncology services coordinator, a newly created post at Bermuda's only general hospital, the King Edward Hospital VII Memorial Hospital. She was the sole person directly involved with cancer care at the Hospital and acted as the tumor registrar, secretary to the weekly tumor conference, administrator of chemotherapy, and counselor to the patients and nurses. At that time it was estimated (but not documented) that approximately 50% of all cancer patients were dying within 1 year of diagnosis.

In 1980, Mrs. Soares traveled to England to observe and gain knowledge in palliative care. She visited several locations, including St. Joseph's Hospice and the Royal Marsden Hospital in London. She readily absorbed the concept of palliative care, having taken it as part of her own philosophy during nursing school days.

Upon her return to Bermuda, Mrs. Soares was dismayed to realize that, with very few exceptions, no one was remotely interested in hearing about care of the dying. She was instructed not to discuss death with patients. Only one or two physicians permitted Mrs. Soares to visit their hospitalized cancer patients. In speaking to ward nurses, she learned there were between 20 and 30 such dying patients who were spending long periods of time in the hospital, many abandoned and neglected by their families. With absolutely no community support system in existence, it was too expensive to keep patients at home. There was considerable fear of death in general, and families were simply unable or unwilling to care for their loved ones in the home setting.

"Cancer" was a word hardly spoken aloud in the community. Patients were isolated for fear of contamination, and families were even afraid to use the same utensils. Patients were denied the affection they so desperately needed from loved ones who, in their ignorance, feared that a kiss or any physical contact would result in their contracting the dreaded disease. After a few months and a few prayers, a giant step forward was taken when Mrs. Soares was finally given permission to visit hospitalized cancer patients with the view of doing all she could to help them.

# THE BEGINNING OF P.A.L.S.

To comfort those patients unable to return home, nursing friends were approached who, hopefully, would volunteer their time to sit and talk to patients, perhaps feed them, read to them, and generally keep them company. One of those first volunteers offered to sit with a lady whose life was rapidly drawing to a close. It was not until it was too late to make other arrangements that Mrs. Soares realized with horror that the volunteer happened to be the wife of a funeral director, whose visit could easily have been misinterpreted!

However, the next morning the patient was still alive, had a big smile on her face and announced "what a wonderful conversation" she had with the volunteer who, as it turned out, did help complete her funeral arrangements, a concern that had weighed heavily on the patient's mind. The volunteer had allowed her to express this worry, and to make her own decisions without persuasion. Fortunately, this first volunteer action proved to be a valuable and meaningful visit.

At this time, very few of the medical fraternity were cooperative. The physicians interpreted death as both a personal failure and a failure of the system. They were not comfortable in confronting the difficult questions put to them by the patients. These questions were more often answered with silence. Details of diagnosis and prognosis were ignored as much as possible. The guidance that we realize today is needed and deserved by each patient was not forthcoming. As in many other places, so it was in Bermuda that the biggest stumbling block to effective medical use of narcotics for pain relief was fear of addiction.

Patients were treated for their serious pain, but often did not respond to the insufficient dose of morphine prescribed. Many died suffering in the belief that nothing more could be done to help them. Mercifully, this is one huge problem that is being recognized and dealt with by most physicians today. We hope that future medical students will graduate with a far deeper understanding and appropriate attitudes toward pain and symptom control, a subject rarely mentioned in medical books until recently.

Later in 1980, some cancer patients were able to return home with a few volunteers checking on them. Assistance for those patients in the community was a priority, but the government-employed district nurses were not comfortable caring for cancer patients, and there were no funds available to employ a special nurse.

The chief medical officer was persuaded to give permission to Mrs. Audra Mitchell, a nurse employed by the Bermuda Tuberculosis, Cancer, and Health Association, to visit cancer patients in the community in addition to her duties of visiting TB patients and checking hotel foodhandlers. The officer limited her cancer patient visits to 3 hours weekly. As anticipated, within a few weeks Mrs. Mithell was spending far more than the permitted time with cancer patients.

When this was realized, the chief medical officer refused to allow her to continue, and it was not until further intense persuasion that she was reinstated.

It was realized that private funds were urgently required by the now budding organization to hire a community cancer nurse. Contact was made with wealthy Hollywood film producer Robert Stigwood, a Bermuda resident at the time. He kindly provided wages for 2 years to employ a part-time nurse. Mrs. Anita Furbert began her duties in February, 1983. Because additional funds would be required for supplies and equipment, Mrs. Soares approached funeral directors. She suggested that they might attempt to persuade families of those deceased cancer patients who had received nursing help gratis to request memorial donations to the organization in lieu of the flowers traditionally sent and often at considerable expense. This idea was accepted by many families and friends, and today accounts for a large portion of our income.

During this time, it was also realized that formal organization of the volunteer program already underway was badly needed, and inquiries were made of other organizations as to how to proceed. Mrs. Margaret Vancrosson thought of the perfect name, P.A.L.S., an acronym for Patients Assistance League and Service.

Mrs. Hilary Soares became Chairman, and Mrs. June Stephens acted as the first Volunteer Coordinator. The first formal minutes of P.A.L.S. were recorded in August, 1980. By the end of 1980, 730 hours had been given by volunteers visiting patients in their homes and in the hospital.

## VOLUNTEER TRAINING

Training sessions continue today for each prospective volunteer. After an initial interview, the prospective volunteer is required to complete an application form, sign a form of confidentiality, and attend the training session before being allowed direct patient contact. The training seminar covers various aspects of P.A.L.S., the definition of cancer, its treatment, and the devastating effects it can have on patients and their families. Other topics include listening skills, the importance of confidentiality, and the role of the volunteer. Additionally, a physiotherapist demonstrates the correct way to assist patients in moving.

Once the seminar is completed, the "PAL" is considered ready for direct patient contact. The volunteers are called upon to do a considerable amount of driving for those patients requiring physician visits, chemotherapy, or blood work at the hospital. A great effort is made to match the personalities and interests of the "PALS" to those of particular patients.

The "PAL" is initially introduced to the patient, usually by the nurse, and then visits the patient regularly, offering friendship and moral support. Often, deep personal and meaningful relationships are formed, especially if the patient is ill for a long time.

Each month, a volunteers' meeting is held to discuss educational topics associated with some aspect of cancer. Today, we have approximately 70 trained and caring volunteers who contribute enormously to the organization. There is considerable difficulty in keeping accurate volunteer statistics, but it is estimated that the volunteers put in an excess of 5,000 hours annually.

Since Bermuda is a small community, volunteers are often recruited through personal friendships, or come to us as people who know and admire our work and wish to be involved to make their own contribution in some way. It is emphasized that a commitment to P.A.L.S. must be given by each volunteer, who is required to provide a minimum of 50 hours annually to the organization. Fortunately, very few applicants are considered unsuitable. The volunteers are supervised by the volunteer coordinator and chief executive officer. If a very ill patient requires several volunteers daily, a roster is drawn up to ensure that the needed hours of companionship are covered. This is deeply appreciated by the loved ones, who are then able to continue with their jobs and attend to other details outside the home. Our volunteers are very aware of patient rights and the fact that we are guests in their homes.

Some volunteers are less comfortable with direct patient contact, but are invaluable in assisting with our regular annual fundraising events and helping in the office. In fact we did not have an office at all until 1984, when the already crowded Bermuda Tuberculosis, Cancer, and Health Association (BTCHA) came to the rescue by kindly providing a tiny cramped room only large enough for one typewriter and our (fortunately petite) volunteer secretary. We eventually managed to squeeze a telephone in also! In 1986, after extensive renovations to the building, BTCHA provided us with a much larger space, including offices and a badly needed storage area. At last, we had a proper home. By 1990, it had become impossible to keep up with the daily routine, and we employed a part-time administrator who is invaluable in the day-to-day operation of P.A.L.S.

## FINANCIAL CONCERNS

Financial challenges must be faced by every charitable organization. It is often the greatest concern faced by executive committees. This is true in the case of P.A.L.S., which provides all nursing and other services entirely without charge. Considerable time and thought is required to ensure that sufficient funds are available to maintain the ever-increasing operating budget.

In 1985, we approached the economic advisor to the Minister of Finance with the request that consideration be given to exempting P.A.L.S. from paying customs duty on items imported for the benefit of cancer patients. With very few exceptions, every solitary item imported into these islands is dutiable (roughly 22%, through this amount varies according to the item. Thankfully, our request was approved, and passed by the legislature, becoming effective in April, 1986. This concession has saved P.A.L.S. thousands of dollars. Bermuda dollars are par with U.S. dollars, and over the years this money has been used effectively within the service.

By 1986, as demands increased, P.A.L.S. was employing one full-time nurse in addition to the original part-time nurse. As the workload continued to grow, the part-time nurse became full-time and it was not long before we realized that even two full-time nurses were not sufficient to maintain the standard of care that had become expected of P.A.L.S. We also realized that P.A.L.S. did not have the necessary funds to employ the additional nurses whom we felt were absolutely necessary to continue giving our patients the highest quality of care and comfort possible. We decided to approach the government again, this time with the request for an annual government grant intended to cover the wages of two additional oncology nurses to match the two nurses already employed by P.A.L.S. Finally, 2 years later, in 1989, with the advice and support of Dr. John Cann, the chief medical officer, our prayers were answered and the government grant became a reality.

With this grant came the huge responsibility of caring for all cancer patients in their homes who wished and required our assistance. It is a responsibility we have always taken very seriously. We are extremely grateful to the government for appreciating our need and granting us this concession, though with the annual increased nursing costs, the 1995 grant fell short of their commitment by many thousands of dollars.

P.A.L.S. expenses are ever-increasing and, in addition to providing wages and supplies, include requests for financial assistance to patients. This assistance ranges from covering the cost of expensive medication not normally available, to paying for the services of a nursing aide, to providing airfares and accommodation for those requiring surgery or treatment abroad. Although chemotherapy is available in Bermuda, radiation is not, as it is felt that a community of this size could not support a radiation unit. Every financial request is considered individually and on its own merits. It is rare if ever, that a bona fide financial request is rejected by P.A.L.S.

For years, P.A.L.S. has been very fortunate in having Mr. John Hill as part of our team in the capacity of treasurer. Mr. Hill's meticulous attention to our finances is certainly a great part of our accountability in the eyes of the public upon whose donations we rely to exist.

Income for P.A.L.S. falls into two major categories, those given as "General Donations" and those given as "Memorial Donations." We also receive funds from many nonunionized workers who elect instead to contribute their mandatory union dues to a charity. We cannot stress strongly enough the vital importance of acknowledging each and every donation, however large or small. In P.A.L.S., no donation is ever considered too small or too insignificant not to warrant a note of grateful thanks. In this respect P.A.L.S. has benefited greatly from 10 years of dedicated work by Mrs. Margaret Tricker serving as memorial secretary. Her hundreds of sensitive and touching acknowledgments of donations are appreciated and valued by the many contributors, and the bereaved families who are informed of them. Every general donation is promptly acknowledged by the president.

Our expenses are ever-increasing and there are always several months in each year when expenses exceed income by thousands of dollars. If donations were not forthcoming, we know that P.A.L.S. would cease to exist. Of these essential donations, many are very touching. One small boy labored to collect bottles and tins to be recycled. He sent his earning of $3.12 to P.A.L.S. with a charming note written in a shaky hand saying how much P.A.L.S. had helped his beloved Grandpa, and hoping his donation would help us to continue our work. On a recent "tag day" another child, working as a packer at a grocery shop, not only gave his own donation of $1.00 from his earnings, but abandoned his packing job for a few hours to his friends, saying, "He needs the money more than me," and chose instead to proudly help us sell tags! These donations from the heart are very meaningful and important to us, and we value them along with those in the hundreds or even thousands of dollars we receive from others.

We feel strongly that a charity should be seen as making an effort on its own behalf, rather than solely relying on the generosity of others. In this regard, we hold annual fundraising events which include a sponsored walk, an annual fair, a tag day, a slide show, and a fish fry. We also have a successful little cottage industry selling attractive cedar sachets made by volunteers. A local business not only kindly provides the fabric, but also sells the finished product in its shop.

All these events closely involve the volunteers, and to a great extent, many friends of P.A.L.S. There are no prizes for the winners of the sponsored walk, though certificates of participation are given. Everyone who makes the effort to participate is considered a winner, and it is a day when young and old, large and small, and people of all races and religions join hands to support the cancer patients of Bermuda.

## ADMINISTRATION

P.A.L.S. is managed by an executive committee that meets monthly to discuss the affairs of the organization and to make various decisions vital to its continued success. Acting as chairman in a voluntary capacity since 1983, and working out of my own small retail business, I was in constant daily communication with our office administrator via the telephone and fax machine. This arrangement worked well enough for many years, though it was becoming more and more difficult and even inappropriate. Finally it was decided that P.A.L.S. growth and demands required more attention. As a result, another big step forward was taken when I closed my business and was appointed president and chief executive officer in March, 1995. The now enlarged BTCHA kindly provided another small office in their building from which I am able to directly deal with the many responsibilities of the organization. The long-serving vice-chairman, Mrs. Jeanne Edridge, stepped into the vacated chairman's position, and it is felt that we have made the correct decisions with these changes.

## THE NURSES

Looking back, we readily see that the demand for community oncology services has always been present, though unrecognized and unfulfilled until 1980. Since that time, demand has more than tripled. According to statistics, both worldwide and local, the incidence of cancer is not decreasing, and as more and more patients and families become aware of our work, we are receiving more and more referrals.

Some 220 people are diagnosed with cancer in Bermuda annually. This figure also includes the precancers. Approximately 85 patients die each year. Most patients are referred to P.A.L.S. by the oncology department at the hospital. There are also referrals from the physicians, concerned family member, friends, or even the patients themselves. Having made an initial assessment, the nurses visit each patient in their homes as often as they deem necessary. It might only be twice a month or once a week, or might be several times in one day.

Statistics revealing the number of visits made over the course of a year are misleading, as the nurses report their total number of visits, but not units of time. For example, one visit might last 1 hour while another might require 3 hours. In each case, it would be reported as only one visit. In 1994, the four nurses made more than 5,500 such visits. Recognizing the need for additional emotional and bereavement support, P.A.L.S. employed a fifth full-time nurse in 1995, to act as nurse-counselor. Although the four oncology nurses do a great deal of counseling in their everyday duties, it is impossible for them to give every patient, and every family member, especially the children, the intensive counseling so many desperately need in their sad and trying circumstances.

P.A.L.S.' executive committee is also well aware of the importance of keeping our nurses informed and up to date with the latest trends and procedures in oncology care. To accommodate this requirement, each nurse in turn since 1987 has attended educational courses abroad in the United Kingdom, the United States, and Canada. In this way, they learn of current nursing procedures and new ideas. It is rewarding for us all when the nurses return from their courses feeling confident and happy about our work here after interacting with their peers from other areas of the Western world.

Bermuda is small enough so that all our nurses, acting essentially as nurse practitioners, have almost instant access to the physicians. The P.A.L.S. nurses attend to the total care of their patients, calling upon all the available resources necessary. Those resources include Meals on Wheels, government nurses' aides, social assistance, the government psychologist, and Child and Adolescent Services, to name a few.

In the beginning, the P.A.L.S. nurses were obliged to use their own private cars for transportation. Gradually we have built up a fleet of four minivans, all of them donated, and all of them proudly displaying the P.A.L.S. logo and name of the donor. The patients are divided up geographically in order to keep driving to a minimum, and each nurse carries a great deal of needed supplies in her van.

The hospice coordinator, staff of six registered rurses and six nursing aides are supported by volunteers, who assist in many ways, including sitting with patients and preparing and serving meals. A government reinsurance program covers the daily cost of patients admitted to Agape House. Those not covered by this program come in under the hospital's indigent fund.

With the fifth P.A.L.S. nurse in place, we feel that at present we are able to meet the needs of the cancer patients at home; these patients now number well over 100 on any given day. Presently, we find there is little difficulty in encouraging people to take advantage of our program, though in the past some patients would not even permit the P.A.L.S. van to be seen on their property for fear the neighbors would know of their diagnosis of cancer.

## THE CHALLENGE OF AIDS

In 1987 came the reality of the dreaded H.I.V. virus. At first there was considerable concern regarding the safety of the nurses exposed to patients suffering from Acquired Immune Deficiency Syndrome. We realized very quickly that we could neither morally nor professionally refuse to care for AIDS patients suffering from cancer. Like care providers around the world, we sought instructions in the correct procedures to safely care for these patients safely and effectively.

In 1991, after much heated public controversy regarding a suitable location, the Bermuda Hospitals Board opened Agape House, a 12-bed hospice originally intended for AIDS patients. Located within the hospital grounds, it shares the services of the hospital and is an attractive option for cancer patients if circumstances make it impossible for them to remain at home during the last few weeks or days.

Unfortunately, to some extent there still remains the erroneous belief that a P.A.L.S. van always symbolizes imminent death. This, however, is definitely not the case, as P.A.L.S. exists to assist any cancer patient in any stage of his/her disease. We actively promote "living with cancer," making every day count and enjoying life on our beautiful island to the fullest extent possible. We frequently have patients who are treated, cared for, and are well enough to be discharged from our service. Surprising as it may sound, some patients will do all they can to remain on our books, even though they are considered physically well and free of disease! This is a result of the special bond of trust and friendship that has developed between the nurse and/or volunteer.

P.A.L.S. differs somewhat from the usual hospice in that we do not restrict our patients to those with a life expectancy of 6 months or less. We offer care and emotional support to all cancer patients needing help from diagnosis, to discharge or until the close of life. To quote one of our nurses: "Every once in a while you get a patient who is a gift. You learn so much from that patient. She touched me so much with her wonderful outlook on life." And from another P.A.L.S. nurse: "It is wonderful that P.A.L.S. decisions are made instantly. There is little red tape regarding financial requests—it is like a dream." Yet another nurse recently expressed her thoughts: "I think P.A.L.S. is doing a fantastic job and maybe doing it better than anywhere else in the world. It is the most satisfying job I could do."

## LOOKING BACK

I believe that among P.A.L.S.' most significant accomplishments is the recognition, acceptance, respect, and reliance we now receive from the physicians and health care professionals of these islands. Almost the entire community associates the word "cancer" with P.A.L.S. Over the years, we have been able to cope with the increasing demand by employing additional nurses before a crisis situation was allowed to happen. We have managed to gather a band of special and caring volunteers upon whom we can rely. P.A.L.S. has played a major role in helping to unite families within their own homes.

P.A.L.S. has also acquired a great deal of equipment, including wheel chairs, walkers, electric beds, commodes, oxygen concentrators, and suction machines, all of which are available to our patients at no charge whatsoever. Much of this equipment has been donated by other charitable groups, businesses, or individuals.

Every P.A.L.S. patient receives the same care, the same dedication, and friendship regardless of their financial circumstances. Color, creed, or race has never been a consideration for admission to our program.

Parents and children have become closer to each other in their mutual desire to do all they can to help a loved one. At last death is beginning to be recognized as a part of life, and many more families are finding it easier to talk about death and face the issues they have always avoided as much as possible.

## LOOKING AHEAD

We strongly believe that however good a job everyone tells us we are doing, it is vital that we must continue to strive to maintain the highest quality of care possible. We hope to develop an even stronger multidisciplinary team to better enhance cancer care in Bermuda. We would like to play a greater part in public education regarding early diagnosis leading to more cures. We are at present actively pursuing plans to enlarge our premises. Additional office space is needed again, and there is an urgent need to increase our overcrowded storage area.

We would like to expand the role of the volunteer to include increased appropriate limited respite care. We would also like to increase volunteer hours to meet the present, growing, and anticipated needs, utilizing volunteer time as effectively as possible. We hope to increase even further public awareness of our program and of the vital need for ongoing, private, and public financial support. The area most in need of research and evaluation is improvement of our own statistics. Our recent acquisition of a computer should be very useful in this effort. Above all, we intend to continue to provide cancer patients at home with the most appropriate, most effective, most efficient, and highest quality of care possible.

## POINTS TO CONSIDER IN DEVELOPING A HOSPICE PROGRAM TODAY

Because of recent trends and worldwide media and journalistic coverage, those persons considering the development of a hospice and palliative care program may already be a few steps ahead of the initial difficulties experienced by P.A.L.S. and other efforts that struggled on unfamiliar ground years ago. Public awareness has heightened the recognition and acceptance of the overwhelming need to provide similar programs available to all people, which should make the task of setting up programs a little easier.

Even so, newcomers will undoubtedly face many challenges. They would be well advised to plan very carefully before proceeding. Consideration must be given to all aspects of their dream. They should target the medical fraternity and other people whose understanding and cooperation is essential.

It is vital to choose nurses very carefully. Nurses may have all the credentials on paper, but it is just as important that they must be compassionate and possess the dedication "to go the extra mile." They must impress upon all those involved with their program the importance of being a team member, and of having the desire to do their best for each and every patient without exception.

## SOME FULFILLING REWARDS OF HOSPICE WORK

In the course of our work, we have had many memorable experiences and powerful impressions, mostly from the patients themselves. Their bravery and inner strength in facing months and years of often painful and unpleasant treatments and side effects is extraordinary to witness. To answer those who say they could "never do this work because it is too depressing" my answer is always the same. "I do not deny that we often experience very sad times; that we have felt the deep loss of countless friends over the years; but the fulfillment we feel and spiritual uplifting we experience is at least equal to the comfort we can give our patients."

# 7

# The Royal Victoria Hospital Palliative Care Service: A Canadian Experience

Balfour Mount, M. D.

## GENESIS

How did it all start? "One thing just led to another" characterizes the process, an unfolding of events colored by synchronicity and a sense of the inevitable. But to begin at the beginning:

In January, 1973, a group of us agreed to give an evening seminar on death and dying at a local church. During the planning session, a surgical colleague commented that instead of simply exchanging anecdotes about inadequate terminal care, we should do a study to determine how patients really die at our McGill teaching hospital. A research grant was obtained. The resulting studies (Ad Hoc Committee on Thanatology, 1973; Mount, Jones, & Patterson, 1974) documented the fact that our respected Montreal institution had a serious problem.

The Royal Victoria Hospital (RVH) assessment of care received by terminally ill patients involved both quantitative and qualitative strategies. The two main conclusions of these studies were (1) care of the dying was seriously deficient, and

(2) we were generally unaware of the suffering experienced by these patients and their families.

A series of case studies compiled by a medical student research assistant provided illuminating insights into the problems faced by our patients. Nine of these disturbing accounts of inadequate care were included in the final report to the Hospital Board. One follows.

> Mrs. P. was admitted with symptomatic advanced retroperitoneal fibrosarcoma. Physical examination revealed a pleural effusion, hepatomegaly, ascites, and peripheral edema. On the day of admission she stated, "Why are doctors so frightened by death? Why don't they talk to their patients about it? Can't they help people through their dying? They tried to tell my husband [my diagnosis] 3 years ago, but his English isn't so good. It was only a few weeks ago when I found out. It was in the clinic and I finally got the intern to tell me I had cancer, but I never could get him to tell me how I'll do.
>
> If only we had known 3 years ago. We'd been in Canada 38 years. We've worked hard and saved for a trip home to Norway, and to see the grandchildren in England. Three years ago we could have gone. Now we shall never go. . . . I'm not afraid to die. It's part of life. . . . No, I don't go much for religion, really. Still, there must be something after death. . . . I want to be with my son again. He was lost a few years ago.
>
> During her admission Mrs. P.'s condition improved and she was discharged. On a followup visit she was accompanied by her husband, who requested a private interview with the doctor. After a wait of an hour, the doctor confronted him.
>
> "There is nothing we can do medically. We can only keep her comfortable. I'm sorry, but this is it. Is there anything else you would like to know?"
>
> The meeting lasted less than 2 minutes. With his voice cracking, the husband left the room. Upon meeting the student interviewer, he stared blankly; "You doctors really don't understand."
>
> The doctor's entry in Mrs. P.'s clinic chart stated in effect that the situation had been explained in detail to the patient's husband and that all supportive measures had been taken.

It was 1973—what recommendations could we make to improve the lot of our dying patients? While pondering that question, I read Elisabeth Kubler-Ross' (1969) landmark book, *On Death and Dying*. I was struck by the similarity of her observations—the blocked communications, inadequate symptom control, isolation, fear, and distrust—to those now documented at our hospital, and, indeed, to my own experience as a cancer patient a decade earlier. I noted Kubler-Ross's reference to Dr. Cicely Saunders and her work with the dying in England. Flipping to the bibliography I found seven articles listed under "Saunders," dating from 1959. Clearly, Kubler-Ross and Saunders were way ahead of the rest of us.

On an impulse, I asked the overseas telephone operator for St. Christopher's Hospice in London. There was a little money left in the grant; it could pay my way to London to see this "home for the dying," that Saunders had created. And while in London I could take in some theater. Superb!

I remember being impressed by the unique blend of friendliness and efficient professionalism conveyed by the voice that answered, "St. Christopher's Hospice." I asked for Dr. Saunders, explaining that I was calling from McGill University in Montreal. In moments a second voice intoned, "Dr. Saunders." I briefly recounted the story of our study and asked whether I might visit. The reply was immediate. "I am on my way to lunch. I can't possibly think of such things right now! Call me back in an hour!" I was delighted by her response!

Things didn't go as I'd planned on the return call either. After listening silently to my request, Dr. Saunders asked, "When do you want to come? "Well, I hate to sound so American," I replied, "but I was wondering about next week?" Once again the response was immediate. "I know you! You want to come to London, see some plays and then have a quick look around here. Well, it won't do! I'll tell you what; leave your wife at home, plan to stay for a week, be prepared to roll up your sleeves and get to work, and we'll have you!"

I awakened from a deep sleep two nights before the flight, suddenly aware of a problem. I was off to England, but to see what? As a surgical oncologist I could think of 50 reasons why putting dying patients together was a bad idea! If by chance I was wrong, I'd have to see it to believe it. It was clear to me that I needed to take along a camera, or my colleagues at the Royal Vic would be no more convinced than I. Not owning a camera, I borrowed one en route to the airport.

## A WEEK AT ST. CHRISTOPHER'S

The week spent at St. Christopher's was life-transforming. Over the ensuing decades, several aspects of that first visit continue to stand out vividly:

- The use, in pain relief, of individually optimized doses of opioids, dispensed as the "Brompton Mixture," at intervals dictated by the pharmokinetics of the opioid being used;
- The medical management of malignant bowel obstruction;
- The aura of peace, purpose, welcome, and security that permeated every corner;
- The reassuring evidence of an efficient, skilled, and wonderfully caring team that was physician-rich, including, as it did, doctors Saunders, Tom West, Mary Baines, Colin Murray Parkes, and Therese Vanier, not to mention the young research fellow, Robert Twycross;
- The attention given to the complex needs of family members;

- The perceptive assessment of psychosocial and spiritual issues, as part of an expanded health care mandate that aimed at the alleviation of suffering rather than simply fighting disease;
- Home care competence;
- Respect for the patient and family as teachers; and
- Incorporation of research and teaching as essential components of care for this forgotten patient population.

In keeping with the spirit of hospitality that was so evident, I was invited to the Director's office for a drink as the afternoon of my first day wound to a close. "What will you have? We have sherry and Scotch. I am having Scotch." Deeply moved by all I had seen, and feeling unduly close to my gracious host, I found myself awkwardly asking how she preferred to be addressed. Peering over her Scotch she fixed me with a penetrating gaze. "My friends call me Cicely." Then, sensing the wheels spinning in my amply impressed brain, she added: "Steady, boy, I said my *friends* call me Cicely. Others call me Dr. Saunders!"

It seemed a lifetime later when, photos of my newly acquired patient teachers having been taken, I bid farewell to my mentors and received an unexpected parting gift: "You may call me Cicely."

## BACK TO THE ROYAL VIC

One thing troubled me about St. Christopher's as a model for transforming the dreadfully inadequate care of the dying that encircled the globe. This outstanding multimillion pound institution met the needs of a small neighborhood in southeast London, centered on the hospice and having a radius of approximately 5 miles. It seemed unlikely that health care could afford a sufficient number of hospices to meet the needs of the 80% of society who die in institutions. Someone had to attempt to duplicate the full St. Christopher's Hospice model—home care, inpatient beds, bereavement support program, consult service to the other hospital wards, and research and training—in the context of the "high-tech" institutions responsible for the care of patients with life-threatening disease. Cicely expressed doubt regarding this proposal, noting the divergency between the goals of the two types of institutions. Nevertheless, the recommendations of our research committee were now clear (Mount, 1976).

The Royal Victoria Hospital Board received our report of deficient care with concern, and was greatly impressed by the slides that had been taken illustrating patient and family comfort at St. Christopher's. It was a marvelous example of Cicely's dictum, "Let the patients do the teaching." The slides had a similar impact at Grand Rounds on all the major clinical services. The Board accepted in principle the recommendation that a specialized service for the terminally ill be established as a 2-year pilot project.

The term "hospice" has pejorative connotations in French and Spanish. What, then, could we call the proposed program? The answer occurred to me one morning while I was shaving. "There are Dialysis Units, Coronary Care Units, Intensive Care Units . . . why not 'Palliative Care Units'? PCU? Perfect!" This designation offered a neutral and somewhat ambiguous alternative. "To palliate" had its origins in the Latin *pallium*, or cloak. This term initially meant to conceal or hide. More recently, however, it had come to mean "to mitigate the suffering of; to ease."

While I was delighted with the term, my British colleagues were less impressed. One letter from Robert Twycross, on behalf of others, was particularly strident in opposing this new term. Characteristically, some time later I received a followup letter from Robert declaring his change of mind on etymological grounds. "Palliative Care Unit" was a go, at least as an acceptable term.

A great distance separates "agreement in principle" and actual program development. The whole thing might have ended before it started, had it not been for an unexpected twist of fate. Nursing salaries at that time were considerably lower in the province of Quebec than in neighboring Ontario. The nurses first negotiated, then demonstrated, and finally struck—but all to no avail. Next, they started to leave the province. This resulted in bed closures, including the Royal Vic's internationally respected Metabolic Investigation Unit.

A golden opportunity! Would the hospital agree to a 2-year experimental trial of palliative care in this vacated 12-bed unit, if we could attract nurses to staff the new program? The hospital would. And the nurses came. They came not only from within Quebec, but from Ontario as well, an early indication of the existing dissatisfaction with traditional care and the great appeal of palliative care.

It is difficult from this vantage point, more than two decades later, to appreciate the radical newness of the proposal that faced the Royal Vic. A hospital whose considerable reputation had been forged through excellence in the science and technology of medicine was being asked to undertake what appeared to be a loss of acute care beds, and all in the interest of those for whom "nothing more can be done."

"Besides," a medical oncologist commented during the meeting of the Council of Physicians and Dentists convened to determine whether the proposal should be passed, "We already give this sort of care to our patients. Furthermore, all my patients are dying. If this [the PCU] were to happen, I would lose all my patients. We do not need the proposed service." A critical moment.

Support for the proposal came from only a few key figures. To many others, the concept seemed antithetical to the hospital mandate.

I responded, "I am surprised, 'Tom,' that you would make such a comment without having read the Committee report. Did you read the report?" To his embarrassment he was forced to admit in front of all assembled that he had not. "Tom" sat down, silenced. My confrontational question had been a calculated risk, but a fairly safe one. His patients were the subject of several of the case studies in the Committee report. While others would not realize this, he would have, had he read the document. The day had been won.

Within 6 months, the new programs had proven itself clinically. Within 2 years, its effectiveness was supported by published data (Melzack, Ofiesh, & Mount, 1976; Mount, 1976; Royal Victoria Hospital Palliative Care Services, 1976) and by an International Seminar on Terminal Care, November 3–5, 1976. This was the first of the biennial International Congress series that has continued over the ensuing two decades. The first seminar featured Dr. Saunders, Dr. Kubler-Ross, Dr. Sylvia Lack, the current and former McGill Deans of Medicine, and The Royal Victoria Hospital Directors of Oncology, Surgery, Obstetrics/Gynecology, Psychiatry, and Professional Services, as well as members of the RVH PCU team. The future of the Palliative Care Service (PCS) was assured.

## A SENSE OF "GIVENNESS"

A recounting of these early days of the RVH PCU seems to me incomplete without reference to an overarching phenomenon that accompanied these experiences. Cicely has referred to her hospice quest as "a vocation from God" (Kastenbaum, 1993). While for many, such a claim must seem a comment appropriate only to an earlier period of history, I suspect that others will share my feeling of identifying with her experience, if not her penchant for frank talk when dealing with matters spiritual. The fact is that the last two decades have been colored by many instances that were characterized by a sense of "givenness." These moments are hard to describe, harder still to explain, unless one simply accepts them as manifestations of the spiritual: the mystery at the heart of meaning and existence. I have already referred to my nocturnal awakening to the need of a camera and the synchronicity of the nursing exodus that enabled the PCU to come into being. Two other examples of this phenomenon stand out.

Flying over the Atlantic on my return from that first visit to St. Christopher's in September, 1973, I wondered whom one could call on to develop the medical component of such a program. To my surprise, the question had no more than taken shape in my mind then the answer presented itself as well—Dr. Ina Ajemian. The surprising aspect of this thought lay in the fact that I did not know Ina well. We had met socially once or twice through my passing acquaintance with her husband, but we had had no contact professionally. Furthermore, Ina was a family physician by training, and family physicians did not have admitting privileges at the Royal Vic.

There was no palliative care program to invite her to join, and there certainly was no identified income for her, but I decided to trust my intuition, and phoned Ina the next morning. I shall never forget her comment once I had reminded her who I was and had told her why I was calling. (This involved a description of St. Christopher's, my reason for being there, my fantasy that the Vic needed a similar program, and the thought that she would be admirably suited to such a challenge.) She replied, "I find it strange that you should call right now. Over the last few days I have had the most powerful sense that I should be open to changing what I am doing. I shall take this very seriously."

Ina became the founding physician in charge of medical care on the PCU, in the process dropping to approximately one-fifth of her previous income. Later she became director of the program, until her departure in 1993 to head the Palliative Care Service at Dalhousie University.

About 3 months after the Palliative Care Service started, I was awakened unexpectedly from a deep sleep to find myself engulfed by feelings of anxiety and aware that we were "skating on thin ice." We had no medical "bench strength" should anything happen to Ina. Indeed, should the housekeeper who helped with her children become ill, we would be in serious trouble. Once again, no sooner had I articulated the question then the answer presented itself. In this instance the answer was John Scott, a young family physician just out of internship. This idea was certainly unexpected. I had been introduced to John only once, perhaps a year earlier. We had not really spoken.

I called John early the next morning. My explanation regarding who I was and why I was calling seemed tortuous and implausible, even to me. What must he be thinking? His reply was immediate and to the point. "I find it strange that you should call right now. I am sitting here reading about the calling of Abraham. I shall have to take this call seriously." John joined the PCS and developed the Consult Service and Home Care Program. He later studied theology, then epidemiology. Currently he directs the regional Palliative Care Service for the University of Ottawa.

## SUPPORTERS AND DETRACTORS

The paradoxes of palliative care lie at the root of much of the resistance we faced in the early days of the program. For example, many feared that a palliative care ward might ghettoize the dying. In fact, however, it is on the acute treatment ward, where their presence is an indictment of the system, that the dying are likely to be isolated and ignored. Furthermore, many felt that a PCU might promote a preoccupation with death. Actually, effective symptom control, and the presence of those who are there because they *choose* to care for the dying, frequently produces a liberation that enables the patients to focus on living and the quality of each day rather than on dying. With time, these realities of hospice life became evident, and antagonism lessened.

Nothing wins hospice care more staunch supporters than the evidence of clinical competence. The Chief of Surgery at the Vic, hitherto a bemused on-looker, referred one of his patients to the PCU. A man in his early fifties, the patient had been suffering severe intractable pain for several months, pain that the Chief of Surgery's best efforts had not alleviated. Forty-eight hours later, as we passed each other in the hall, the surgeon commented enthusiastically, "Oh, Bal— that girl is *very* good!" It took some time to realize that he was speaking about Ina. His patient's pain had been controlled and we had won an ardent ally. Bad news spreads quickly. Happily, so does news of the unexpected alleviation of suffering.

Throughout the initial years of the RVH PCU, Drs. Saunders and Kubler-Ross lent generous support with frequent visits. On one such visit, Dame Cicely and I were in the PCU when a large dog, the beloved "key person" of one of the patients, ambled across the hall and into his room. "You see that dog?" I commented nonchalantly, with no little pride, "Part timber wolf." Cicely's only reply was an acknowledging nod and a quiet, "Hmmmmm," as if she had timber wolves at St. Christopher's every day, or at the very least wasn't surprised to encounter one on a ward here in the colonies. I had forgotten the incident when a short time later I received a cryptic note from Cicely. "Have just had baby elephant." It seems that an employee of a traveling circus had been admitted to St. Christopher's, and a young elephant, with whom he had developed a close bond, had come for a visit. I wrote back a one line reply. "Shall never try to 'one-up' you again!"

When starting the PCU, we had anticipated that our greatest support would come from the internists in the hospital, and that we would encounter less tolerance and understanding from the surgeons. This was not the case. It was instead our surgical colleagues who were most supportive, understanding of our goals, and ready to refer. The internists tended to find the palliative care service more problematic, apparently having trouble accepting the possibility that they might not be delivering adequate palliative care themselves.

At the very beginning, support came from many quarters. A local charitable foundation gave the first start-up grant. Key figures at McGill University lent their encouragement. Members of the public, on hearing of our work through the media, pitched in. Hospital employees at all levels throughout the Royal Vic became advocates. For example, when the hospital unions went on strike during a particularly bitter support, they barred volunteer replacement workers from all floors except the Palliative Care Unit. Most critically, support came from our patients, their families and friends, and from our own families. The recognition that success at the Royal Vic would influence the care of the dying internationally fueled and sustained effort at a fever pitch. Our families demonstrated remarkable patience and understanding.

As the years passed, our referral base broadened, with consultations relating to an increasingly diverse range of clinical problems and at progressively earlier points in the disease trajectory. In recent years, antagonism has generally risen in relation to two issues: (1) philosophical-opposition to housing a palliative care program in the high-cost, highly specialized environment of a tertiary care hospital, and (2) competition for scarce resources. As the physician-in-chief put it during one memorable phone call, "Well, Bal, with the impending budget cuts I have to close either the Coronary Care Unit, the Dialysis Unit, one of the two remaining Medical Clinical Teaching Units at the Vic, or the Palliative Care Unit. What would you suggest I do?"

# FINANCIAL REALITIES

Palliative care as practiced by the Royal Vic team includes a daily patient/family census of 80–100 on home care, another 20–30 followed by the Consultation Service on the active treatment wards of the hospital, and 16 in the Palliative Care Unit. Additionally, there is bereavement support for the most needy families during the first year following their loss. The origins of PCU referrals are: Medicine, 38%; Surgery, 35%; Gynecology, 8%; Oncology Clinics, 5%; Neurology/Neurosurgery, 4% and all other services, 10%.

The costs involved in caring for these patients do not, in general, represent additional expenses, since our clients are Royal Vic patients who would be dying on our wards in any case. Palliative care groups these patients together, improves their care, avoids admission for many who are able to be at home, and shortens the length of stay when admission is required, resulting in an increased availability of medical and surgical active treatment beds. Between 15–20% of those in the RVH PCS home care program die at home. The need for an effective palliative care service to maximize the effectiveness of bed utilization becomes increasingly evident as health care budgets tighten.

A striking example of the critical role played by the PCS was precipitated by the recent closure of four PCU beds because of budget constraints. This 25% reduction in the number of PCU beds led to an immediate increase in the number of patients waiting for a palliative care bed on a given day. The usual waiting list of 2–4 patients increased to as many as 18. This extra pressure was felt most severely in the hospital's Emergency Department. The disproportionate increase in the number of patients waiting for a bed compared to the number of beds closed is understood to reflect the degree to which patient care and the flow of patients through the system depend on the availability of a number of beds that is close to the existing need of the institution. A month after the bed closure, an anonymous donor in the community reopened the beds. This action resulted in an immediate return to the previous norm of 2–4 patients waiting. The entire process of reducing, then restoring, the beds demonstrated both community support and the impact of palliative care on overall health care dynamics.

Palliative care patients are among the sickest in any hospital and have great nursing care needs. As measured by the PRN needs assessment system (EROS, 1990), PCU patients have a mean of 9.0 hours of nursing care needs per day as compared with 6.4, 5.6, and 5.1 hours for medical, surgical, and geriatric ward patients, respectively. Our experience suggests that quality care can be delivered without significant increase in expenditure, in spite of the need for a high nurse/ patient ratio. (This ratio is intermediate between the levels needed for a general medical ward and for intensive care nursing.) Comparing costs for PCU, medical, and surgical wards, respectively, the total costs per patient day are $191, $217, and $191. Annual direct costs per bed are $61,675; $74,697; and $62,376 (McGill Soins Palliatifs, 1993).

Quality palliative care demands the involvement of a physician-rich team. The mechanism of physician reimbursement thus becomes a determining factor in the provision of this care. The nature of the care involved dictates that fee-for-service reimbursement generates a very small income. It is therefore critical to make available a fair salary for doctors who practice palliative medicine. Such a system became available in Quebec soon after the opening of the PCS, thus enabling the development of a strong physician component on the clinical team. Now, however, 20 years later, budgets are tightening further, and the survival of this mechanism of reimbursement in all likelihood depends on Palliative Medicine becoming a recognized specialty in Canada, as is already the case in the United Kingdom, Australia, and New Zealand.

A portion of the PCS costs are not covered by existing hospital budgets, including the psychologist (21 hours per week); music therapist (24 hours), occupational therapist (18 hours), volunteer coordinator, bereavement service coordinator, and one secretary. In addition, research personnel are not funded through existing hospital or university budgets, nor do the physicians have nonclinical funding to support research time. As a result, the annual PCS funding shortfall is approximately $200,000 (Canadian). Public financial support is thus essential.

## VOLUNTEERS

Volunteers enrich the lives not only of our patient/family clients but of their colleagues on the PCS team. They bring creativity, freshness, wisdom, and a deep humanity born out of a wealth of life experience. Volunteers contribute endless hours of skilled listening, afternoon concerts, happy hour, fundraising, telephones answered, bed baths and whirlpool baths, massages, bereavement support, cups of tea, hours of committee, and office work. The list goes on— leadership in every sphere, grace upon grace upon grace.

As we mark our 20th anniversary, we have just hired our third Director of Volunteers. This remarkable continuity—only two Directors in two decades—has been a great help in establishing a strong team numbering approximately 100 active volunteers at any time. We have never actively recruited volunteers. They come by self-selection from all walk of life, having heard of the PCS through friends, relatives, or the media. Frequently, the experience of a personal loss has attuned them to the work.

Volunteers are screened by the coordinator in in-depth interviews prior to commencing their work with us. They become acclimatized to the PCU through the buddy system, working alongside an experienced volunteer. With experience, volunteers may be selected to join the Consult, Home Care, or Bereavement Support teams. An annual 16-hour training course is mandatory for volunteers and recommended for nonvolunteer staff. Volunteers are also expected to participate in continuing education and staff support programs.

## GROWTH: FROM RVH PCS TO PALLIATIVE CARE MCGILL

In 1991, McGill University developed a centralized Department of Oncology that brought together relevant basic science and clinical programs from all McGill-affiliated institutions. At the recommendation of the Dean of Medicine, Palliative Care McGill (PCM) was named as one of the divisions, indicating the university's intent that standards of palliative care should be equal across all McGill hospitals. There was agreement that the terms of reference of PCM would not be limited to oncology, but would also include nonmalignant terminal illness.

Over the ensuing years, PCM has expanded to include programs in the community and in 10 hospitals. Although the individual programs are operating at widely differing stages of development, each with its growing pains and challenges, the total network provides a critical mass that facilitates teaching and research and provides improved care to a significantly increased number of patients and their families.

## IN RETROSPECT AND PROSPECT

The editors of this volume have asked us to reflect on our achievements and failures, our aspirations and concerns as we look to the future. Looking back over the past 20 years, we envision a sea of faces—the men, women, and children who as patients or family members have been our teachers. What lessons have they taught? They have challenged us to develop more effective symptom control, to reach a deeper understanding of the rich complexity of human wholeness, to give renewed attention to the multiple contributors to healing—physical, psychosocial, and spiritual—and to a broader health care mandate that moves beyond fighting disease to embrace the alleviation of suffering.

As we look to the future, we are focused on a spectrum of goals. In the clinical sphere, our goal is to define new patterns of delivering home-based and institutional palliative care that remain faithful to Dame Cicely's concepts, while observing the ever-increasing limitations imposed by financial constraints that challenge the international community. We look forward to the recognition of Palliative Medicine as a new discipline in Canada and to participating in the development of the associated training programs, as well as the maturing of a Canadian network for palliative care research.

What of our accomplishments to date? We believe the decision taken at the Vic to integrate hospice beds, consultation services, home care, bereavement followup, research, and teaching in a tertiary care hospital was of fundamental importance. We relish the challenge of being catalysts for whole person care in a center striving for excellence in academic medicine. We take satisfaction in the consult from the "cath lab" for music therapy to assist the anxious young woman who is about to undergo cardiac catherization; in the consult from the ICU to assist their staff in explaining the condition of a brain-dead father to a little boy; and in collaborating with our oncology colleagues by measuring quality of life during a trial of high-dose chemotherapy for women undergoing bone marrow transplantation for breast cancer. We take satisfaction in our early inclusion in the management of most oncology patients treated at the Vic, and our participation in patient care and teaching on the medical and surgical wards. *We have shown that hospice can be integrated into the warp and woof of health care and academic medicine.*

Do we have regrets? "Of him to whom much is given, much shall be required." We were handed a unique opportunity by a visionary hospital and medical school. How did we measure up? We see the faces of all those whose suffering we failed to control; the opportunities missed due to lack of attention to detail; the research left undone. Of course, we could have done more! But we celebrate all that has been done and look to the future with enthusiasm, comforted by Cicely's observation that "the work of building a hospice is never done."

## REFERENCES

Ad Hoc Committee on Thanatology. (1993). *Report to the Royal Victoria Hospital*. Montreal: Author.

Equipe de recherches operationnelles en sant'e. (1990). *System PRN (Projet de recherches en nursing)*. Montreal: Universit'e de Montreal.

Kastenbaum, R. (1993). Dame Cicely Saunders: An *Omega* interview. *Omega: Journal of Death and Dying, 27*, 263–269.

Kubler-Ross, E. (1969). *On death and dying*. New York: Macmillan.

McGill Soins Palliatifs (1993). L'avenir des soins palliatifs au Quebec: Un rapport pour le Ministere de la sant'e et des services sociaux. Monteal: McGill University.

Melzack, R., Ofiesh, J. G., & Mount, B. M. (1976). The Brompton mixture: Effect on pain in cancer patients. *Canadian Medical Association Journal, 115,* 125–129.

Mount, B. M. (1976). The problem of caring for the dying in a general hospital: The palliative care unit as a possible solution. *Canadian Medical Association Journal, 115,* 119–121.

Mount, B. M., Ajemian, I., & Scott, J. F. (1976). Use of the Brompton mixture in treating the chronic pain of malignant disease. *Canadian Medical Association Journal, 115,* 122–124.

Mount, B. M., Jones, A., & Patterson, A. (1974). Death and dying: Attitudes in a teaching hospital. *Urology, 4,* 741–747.

Royal Victoria Hospital Palliative Care Services (1976). *The Palliative Care Service Pilot Project Report.* Montreal: McGill University.

# 8

# Fundacion Omega: Colombia

Isa de Jaramillo

## THE PERSONAL STORY BEHIND FUNDACION OMEGA

I had worked as a clinical psychologist and psychotherapist in Bogata, the capital of Colombia, for more than 15 years. However, one Sunday afternoon early in 1986, the course of my professional life radically changed.

That day I accompanied my husband to visit Teresa, a relative of his, aged 26, who was married and had two daughters, 4 and 2 years of age. She had recently returned from the United States after the failure of her second kidney transplant. During this visit, suddenly all the people disappeared from the room where she lay, and I found myself alone with her. I asked Teresa how she felt. To my surprise, she started to talk and her eyes filled with tears. She told me she was exhausted and tired of suffering.

What made her feel worst, however, was that she had nobody in which to confide. Her mother prodded her to have more faith and to pray. Her mother-in-law told her to be positive towards the illness. Her 31-year-old husband begged her on behalf of himself and their little daughters to try hard and go forth. Her trust moved me deeply, and I suggested it would perhaps be convenient for me to find someone, a psychiatrist, psychologist, or psychoanalyst who could help her in that difficult moment by coming to her house. She accepted. Two hours later I left, worried and deeply committed to my task of finding someone to help her.

For two days, I called all my colleagues, but received only negative responses. Nobody knew what could be done in that case besides giving her antidepressants. A friend of mine, a psychiatrist, told me, "I have a book called *On Death and Dying*, by Kübler-Ross. Why don't you read it, it might be useful." That I did, avidly, and the next day I called Teresa and told her that, having the time, the necessary affection, and my training as a psychologist, I thought I could help her myself. I obviously did not tell her about my failure in getting her a more capable professional to do it. I started visiting her every other day; we talked for hours on end; we shared her fears and her sadness.

Her situation became more critical every day: the pain, the breathing difficulties, the edema, her feeling of isolation despite all the love she received. "I cannot take it anymore . . . I would like to rest." "What do you think is keeping you from doing it?" I asked. "I don't know, perhaps my daughters. Every day that passes is one more day for them." I said, "What would happen if today we spoke about each one of them, about how they are, and perhaps it would help if I should promise you that, once you are no longer here, I would see them, take care of them and supervise their grief process?" Teresa smiled and accepted my proposal with relief. We talked about the girls until darkness set. Next day when I arrived with a bouquet of flowers, I was informed that in the early morning she had gone into a coma. Two days later she died peacefully.

This experience shook me emotionally and made me ponder deeply. It taught me that human beings suffer from solitude, even when there are people around; that sometimes we need someone to sanction our right to die; that when we have some serious unfinished business, we cannot leave; and that we need to share, to cry, and to say goodbye to be able to die better.

Two weeks later, a colleague asked me to help her father who had a lung carcinoma, knowing that I had participated in Teresa's case. When he died, I thought that my background as a psychologist was not enough to continue the exploration of this new professional world that fascinated and excited me. At that time nobody in Colombia could guide me, so I decided to write to Kübler-Ross. She answered, encouraging me to go ahead and invited me to travel, to meet her and assist to her seminars and workshops and to watch her work. I did, and my interest in thanatology grew immensely.

I also went to some other seminars that Concern for Dying had organized in North Carolina, and there I heard William Worden speak and sought contact with others who had been working for years in what was, for me, a new field. I bought books, subscribed to journals, and read all day.

On returning to Colombia, I contacted a new Movement for the Right to Die with Dignity, founded by Beatriz Kopp de Gome. This organization had been established by a board of very important persons who shared that philosophy and were trying to clear the way for the Living Will. In September, 1986, we suffered a very painful family loss, the sudden death of Gabriel, my 15-year-old nephew. Two days later, in a sad and difficult mood, I travelled to Argentina as a guest lecturer at the First International Meeting on Palliative Care to speak about my experience with terminal patients and the right to die. There I met the other two lecturers, Robert Twycross and Geoff Hanks. That was my first contact with hospice or palliative care.

I was astounded on discovering that in other places in the world things could be different and better in regard to dying and this added to the devastating but deeply enriching experience I had when I assisted the gas gangrene-affected survivors of the Armero Volcano Catastrophe to their deaths. I realized that was the new path my professional life should follow, and none other. This prospect frightened, but at the same time, fascinated me. I organized a trip to London, where I finally saw St. Christopher's Hospice and met Dame Cicely Saunders, from whom I received warm and unlimited support. I visited Sobell House, where Robert Twycross patiently and with a deep sense of caring taught me the ABCs of hospice care. Surprised by his secure attitude, I accompanied Geoff Hanks to visit his patients in the Continuous Palliative Care Unit of the Royal Marsden. In a journal, I saw that there was a meeting of the International Work Group on Dying and Death. Not knowing what it was about, I wrote a letter to its president, Thelma Bates, who, after explaining that it was a private group, allowed me to join that meeting. There I met Therese Rando, Charles Corr, Sandy Bertman, Colin Parks, Phyllis Silverman, Betty Davies, and David Adams. All these persons have determined, through their support, wisdom and guidance, the course of palliative care in Colombia.

During the previous semester, some of the colleagues who were close to me had already heard me talking about that new discipline and learning field. My enthusiasm had become contagious, and they had asked me to organize two study groups, with 13 professionals each, to meet weekly so as to read and study the material I had gathered in my trips. On the airplane back from London in July 1987, I decided to establish in Colombia an ambulatory program of hospice care through a foundation that was to be named Omega, because it was a final stop.

At that time I counted on those two groups of professionals to establish this program, and on my family to unconditionally support me, as they always have.


## OMEGA BEGINS

We established the Omega Foundation in August, 1987. A friend of mine, a lawyer, wrote the statutes. Rodrigo, my husband, organized its logistics, and 10 people donated between $5 and $50 each. We rented a house and, introduced by a long article in the most important paper of the country, we opened our doors. Nobody came—only our families and friends.

At the beginning, the team consisted of six psychologists; five are still with Omega 8 years later. They had initially joined me because of our old friendship, one of them being my cousin. They had all had recent personal loss experiences. This group included a psychiatrist (the one who lent me Kubler-Ross's book); two medical doctors who were my friends; two nurses who were working with terminally ill patients; and an anesthesiologist, an old family friend. We continued studying nonstop, and offered the first courses on death, dying, and bereavement ever given in our region.

There was no money to pay wages. Our patients were seen for free, and we survived with the little money made by the courses, whose attendance slowly increased, and the help provided by an executive board coordinated by my husband and friends. Thus, our families and friends were the people who believed in us and made our dream slowly come true.

## RESISTANCE FROM PHYSICIANS AND CULTURAL TRADITION

Physicians were then, and to a certain point still are, indifferent to the situation of the dying person. Psycho-oncology did not exist, and our activities were viewed as threatening by intensive care physicians, oncologists, and other specialized physicians. We visited them, one by one, to explain our philosophy. Most of them expressed admiration towards something they conceived as a rather beautiful charity for the poor. They wished us luck with a smile and little else.

We visited health, educational, religious, and other official institutions and found passive resistance in all of them. We were received everywhere because we had good personal and social references, and also goodwill in our specific fields of previous work. Everywhere, however, our visits concluded without offers of assistance.

A broader resistance was encountered in the death-denying attitude that has become traditional in Colombia. It is useful at this point to review a little of the historical background. The political violence of the 1950s orphaned an entire generation of Colombians. This destructive period has left us with a legacy of resentments, hatred, and poverty. It has also hindered our national development by (a) spawning guerilla movements; (b) serving as a "culture medium" for drug trafficking, thus greatly increasing the crime rate; and (c) resulting in the murder of many political leaders, presidential candidates, judges, magistrates, and military and police officers. Those who try to prevent violence run up against the brick wall of an ever-burgeoning demand for drugs in the United States and Europe. All too frequently, these people themselves become victims of violence.

It is hard to see life as a process in which one's efforts in the present can be expected to yield gains in the future, in a setting in which attempts at positive change seem doomed to failure at the outset. As in any other place in the world where there is a high degree of social mobility and increasing drug consumption, Colombians tend to experience life in terms of the immediate. Values are distorted. Tragedy is transformed into something anecdotal, to be taken for granted in everyday life. Respect is lost; so is any sense of the sacredness of life and the finality of death. In the struggle for survival, the average Colombian is forced to defend him/herself by ignoring the prospects and implications of sudden death. This attitude in turn gives rise to a psychic numbing, a kind of anesthesia of the emotions. Similar responses occur in many other places in the modern world, but it is more common and more intense in Third World countries, and perhaps especially so in Colombia.

More than two-thirds of all deaths among 15–44-year-olds in Colombia are due to violence, whether terrorist, drug-related, or guerrilla. This pattern directly influences the grieving process for survivors. Many persons assisted by Omega have been bereaved by violent deaths. Their reactions range from unremitting anger, to a troubling despair over the authorities' inability to apprehend and punish the guilty parties. Common to these reactions are feelings of impotence, which complicate the task of grieving in a number of ways.

Regarding natural deaths, the first problem faced by a Colombian family when one of its members is in the final stages of an incurable illness is the handling of available information. More specifically, it is the dilemma of whether to reveal or withhold the diagnosis and prognosis. Many people operate on the pretext that telling the truth would be detrimental to the patient's well-being. Families in Colombia tend to be very large, and it is common for one or two members to assume leadership at critical moments. These individuals make decisions about the care of the patient, and act as intermediaries between the physicians and the rest of the family. They also determine which relatives receive complete information, which are given only partial information, and which are given none at all. The group excluded from information frequently consists of elders and children, as well as others who are considered "weak."

The usual procedure is to attempt to shield the patient from his/her own reality. Families go to great lengths to ensure that the patient will receive no information about either the illness or its course. Visits are discouraged. Expressions of affection are avoided because these might prove painful. Verbal exchanges are limited. In this processes, everyone loses. What appears to underlie this phenomenon is a form of magical thinking that is characterized by the simplistic premise that what is not named or expressed ceases to exist. Thus, if there is no aggressiveness, there is no anger. If there are no words, there are no thoughts or feelings. If death is not acknowledged, then it will not occur.

The issue of patient autonomy is overlooked by virtue of this same reasoning. Any desires, preferences, and needs that dying patients might have regarding their care are simply ignored, as if they did not exist; and the same practice applies to the actual circumstances of death.

Place of death is usually determined by economic factors in Colombia. If a family is well off, the patient goes to a private hospital. If not, they usually remain at home. A paternalistic attitude keeps doctors on a pedestal. Their suggestions or decisions are unassailable. This attitude further pre-empts opportunities for decisionmaking by patients and families, reducing their participation to a minimum.

In low-income settings (which include about 80% of the population), the number of patients that physicians must see limits both their availability and the procedures that can be performed. Medical care is at a bare minimum. Many families have only rare and fleeting contact with a physician. For the same reason, pain and symptom control, if it exists at all, tends to be deficient for the homebound terminally ill patient of low or middle income. If they are lucky, a few of the many people who have no regular access to health care services may have occasional help from a neighbor, a relative, or some other doctor that they may happen to know.

In short, between aggressive treatment and the death of the patient, there is a void which nobody fills; and this leads bereaved families to remember the last weeks of the patient's life with pain, anger, and resentment, as a time when they were left to their own devices and denied the adequate medical care to which they felt entitled.

This is the social context of death denial and avoidance that Omega has had to face, a situation that has influenced the hospice project, although, as will be described later, our efforts toward promoting change could be considered slow but successful.

## TERMINALLY III PATIENTS AND THEIR CARE

As this brief history suggests, at the dawn of Omega, there was no conception in Colombia that the patient in a terminal state represented a social problem as well as an individual problem and deserved holistic attention: pain control, and emotional and spiritual support for him and his family.

There was no specialized treatment for the terminally ill. Those with money went to private clinics, where they died undignified and despairing deaths, uninformed, alone, and frightened. Sometimes they were taken home with profound suffering from uncontrolled symptoms, under the care of a physician who was reluctant to visit homes and whose most frequent statement was, "There is nothing else we can do for him (her)." This statement revealed with perfect clarity the physician's incompetence in helping a dying patient. No one would listen to the family, and severe conflicts arose in its midst totally unattended, as death came closer. A Catholic priest would come and give the patient the Anointment for the Sick and offer the family the hope of the forthcoming reunion of this suffering soul with God. This was usually the only acknowledgement and the only act of support received by the patient and family.

Opium derivatives were feared and not used. We might say without exaggeration that many patients were virtually abandoned from a medical point of view long before they died.

Attempts to avoid the impact of death are becoming more common after bereavement as well. Among lower- and middle-class Colombians, it has been common to hold a novena, that is, a mass, for each of the first 9 days following the death of a loved one. This is followed by monthly, then yearly masses, some of them featuring musical groups who serenade the deceased with his/her favorite music. As a sign of mourning, most mourners wear black for a relatively long period of time.

This practice of responding to deaths with rituals and signs of mourning is giving way among affluent Colombians. Strength in adversity is admired, and repressed feelings regarded as a sign of strength. Therefore, crying is to be avoided. The novena, the monthly and yearly masses, and the wearing of black are all being replaced by displays of stoicism which devalue grief and overlook its natural healing powers. These practices include:

- Minimizing the emotional impact of the loss of a loved one by comparing it to the "worse" losses of others;
- Returning as soon as possible to work or to a familiar routine;
- Seeking relief by avoiding memories and other painful reminders of loss through travel or changing residence; and
- Replacing expressions of authentic pain with bravado behaviors that suggest strength and courage.

All these practices are becoming more and more common in Colombia today.

The tendency to deritualize death is largely a defensive response on the part of a society forced to confront multiple deaths by violence. It is also, however, a consequence of U. S. cultural penetration, and goes a long way toward explaining why mental health professionals are seeing more and more instances of unresolved grief, with all the emotional consequences that implies.

## COMMUNITY RESPONSE TO THE FIRST HOSPICE PROJECT

In 1987 the unthought-of happened. A German lady whose mother we had helped during the critical moment of death donated to us $30,000 to be used as a down payment. We purchased a house in a good neighborhood in Bogota, funded by this charitable gift plus a bank loan. This house was to be, then, the first hospice inpatient unit and day care center in Colombia.

At the end of December, the house was severely vandalized and set ablaze. I was personally threatened by furious members of the local community who feared the proximity of dying patients and the possibility that some of them might have AIDS. The reaction was so violent that it became impossible to go on with the project, and we had to abandon it.

We lost the project, the illusion, the money, the house, and part of our team, all within the next 2 months, apparently for different reasons. Half of the team deserted and we remained with no nurses, only one physician, and facing the task of internally rebuilding ourselves and looking for new options and horizons.

We had to confront very hard moments. On January 2, 1988, I went to Asilomar, California, to attend the meeting of I.W.G; I was emotionally devastated and there, all the group, but specially Thelma Bates, John Fryer, Therese Rando, and Steve O'Connor, among other friends, nurtured me with affection and hope to start all over again.

## A NEW DAWN

Omega moved to a tiny apartment (50 sq. meters) without the possibility of seeing patients there for lack of space. We continued the courses on death, dying, and bereavement in an auditorium that was lent to me by the director of a private clinic, a friend of mine. Since that time, all the members of our team have met together on Tuesday afternoons (besides meeting informally several times a week), to share experiences, review cases, and give vent to our reactions and grief due to the death of patients.

At that time our executive board and friends took care of Omega's small expenditures. A friend paid the secretary's monthly fee (she was the only person on salary) and different friends, approached by the Board, took turns at paying our monthly rent. We do not have, and have never had, any steady financial support from any official or private institution.

Even though the situation was deplorable, gratification ensuing from the cases we handled, and the increasing amounts of people attending the courses, gave us strength to go on working.

Nowadays, all the members of our team work part-time at their basic professional activity that constitutes the source of their economic income, and part-time in Omega. The main obstacle to our growth could be summed up in the economic difficulties. We need to establish a more efficient way to pay them adequate wages. A shared commitment to palliative care and the human quality of the team are the cohesive factors that represent for each of us the other fee: the psychic income.

At the present time, each one of us receives a percentage of the income from professional services or courses given during the month. Sometimes the checks are moderately good, but they are very low in relation to what these people deserve as a remuneration for their dedication.

## ACADEMIC OPPORTUNITIES

The School of Psychology at Universidad Javeriana, following my suggestion, opened an optional seminar in thanathology for students in their last semester. I gave the seminar, and that implied the possibility of enlarging our range of action to the academic milieu. Occasionally, the Schools of Medicine invited us to lecture on dying patients.

We began to get more invitations to lecture in different places, and we decided that, so as to nationally broaden the awareness about the importance of palliative care, we should organize an International Symposium. We invited Robert Twycross, Thelma Bates, and Barbara Saunders, and the event was a success. That new project provided excitement and work for many months. In our audience, we had some important local physicians who began to get interested in the dying patient, and then, a year later, we organized a similar event and we brought Mary Vachon and Tony O'Brien; 180 professionals attended each lecture.

The media responded well and echoed our endeavor. Omega became widely recognized nationally.

## THE VOLUNTEERS

We established a volunteer corps with people motivated by our courses and seminars. We tried to implement it, following the example of the Princess Alice Hospice or Sobell House. But even though all these volunteer were very generous and motivated, because of some mistake we have not been able to clearly identify in the team, their aspirations had no boundaries whatsoever. It was not enough for them to help with the administrative part, with the gathering of funds, or with small chores; having assisted as part of their training, with all our courses and seminars—they also wished to perform professional duties and directly help patients and their families. The situation became unmanageable and we were sadly compelled to disband that corps.

## THE INTERDISCIPLINARY TEAM AND, AT LAST,
## ITS OWN HOME

With much effort on our part, on the part of the board, and with the cooperation of persons who had benefited from Omega's services, we bought another house; it has offices and a small lecture room, with maximum capacity for 80–100 persons, so as to correctly establish a Home Care center. We decorated it lovingly, with odds and ends coming from the team members' houses this, complished, we moved into the pleasant, small, and well-cared for house on Kra, 30 No. 89–79 in Bogota.

Slowly the team reestablished itself and reached a better integration. Another physician and another nurse joined it. A well-known physician, Dr. Pedro Bejarano, anesthesiologist and an expert in pain management, came to work with Omega and assumed the task of supervising the work from a medical point of view and make it meet the high standards of the OMS and the NHO. He became, at my side, the medical head of the institution.

All in all, five medical doctors joined us: two general practitioners, and three anesthesiologists who had experience and training in the handling of terminal pain according to the standards of palliative care. We also acquired an occupational therapist and another head nurse, these joined the five psychologists that had been with the team from the beginning, and two more who came motivated by the seminars that are constantly given on thanatology and palliative care. The two general practitioners and these two psychologists entered a 2-year formal training program in palliative care in Omega. Two of them left us later; one of the physicians because he moved away from the city, and one psychologist due to a lack of motivation.

All the team members assist patients at Omega's house until the moment when they can no longer be moved; then we go to their homes, in which case we face the problem of having to cover big distances within the city. Taking into account that Bogota is a city with 6 million inhabitants, very heavy traffic, and enormous distances between one point and another, giving attention to only one patient may take up to 2 or 3 hours.

## CHALLENGES AND IMPROVISATIONS

Even though we have tried to adapt the teachings proven useful elsewhere to our social and cultural environment, we have often faced the necessity of improvising: to look for new, creative solutions for new problems inherent to the social situation of our country.

Thus, for example, we faced the reality of our being the sole institution in Colombia that helps mourners in all the modalities of loss. We found ourselves bound to help people affected by violence, and the hundreds of orphans and widows resulting from guerrilla activity, terrorist bombs, and drug traffic.

We had to design special protocols and strategies to help groups of soldiers and policemen who survived ambushes in which their partners fell; to tend to children, 5 to 10 years old, whose parents had died violently; to organize the way of caring for the 200 families of those who died in an airplane crash; and we were asked by the Military Forces of Colombia to submit a program designed to help the widows and orphans of the dead in action.

Omega was awarded the National Award of Psychology in 1991 for its work, done both in cases of bereavement intervention and in the emotional assistance given to terminally ill patients. In both fields, we were pioneers in Colombia.

## NEEDS AND GOALS FOR FUTURE DEVELOPMENT

We need a more solid economic base, since our income, coming from sales of published material, courses and seminars, and assistance services, permits us to be self-sufficient to survive as an entity; but is still not enough to pay wages.

We would need resources to be able to launch broader and more highly publicized campaigns, and to have the possibility of organizing free courses, which would enlarge the audiences.

Another necessity, also related to economic difficulties, is to finance opportunities for all the members of the team to travel outside Colombia, visiting hospices throughout the world and attending training courses elsewhere; in other words, to enrich their experience.

None of the members of the team have the means to travel on their own. Some of them do not even own a car. With enormous effort, four of the team's professionals have had the chance to visit England and benefit from the ample and generous support that the teachers of palliative care have always offered us. We need this opportunity to be extended to the other eight Omega team members.

## A BOOK ON PALLIATIVE CARE

Following Dr. Bejerano's suggestion, two years ago we wrote and published, *Dying with Dignity: Fundamentals of Palliative Care,* the first text on palliative care written in Spanish. This book contains 28 chapters that cover practically all the basic areas of optimal palliative care. It was written by the 12 members of the Omega Team. The 2,000 books published were financed by a local chemical laboratory and some donations to Omega. This has opened many doors for us on an international level. Now, we continually get letters from interested professionals in the other cities in Colombia and in other countries, such as Argentina, Chile, Panama, El Salvador, Costa Rica. They have all received the book.

## OUR ACHIEVEMENTS

Our most important achievement during these eight years of hard daily work is undoubtedly the creation of a respectable image for Omega and its professionals through the acknowledged quality and efficacy of its services in the different fields: to the dying patients and their families, both in the assistance prior to the death of the beloved person, and after it, during the period of mourning; through professional assistance in tragedies and catastrophes in the country, given the high mortality rate due to violence in Colombia; through the establishment, on the community level, of a popular awareness of palliative care, the rights due to terminally ill patients, the processes of death and mourning, and the role of children facing death in their families; and through the coverage of our seminars and training workshops for professionals in the areas of adequate pain management and other symptoms, patient-physician-family communication, decision-making at the hour of death, and psychosocial aspects of the dying patient and his family, among other topics.

Our statistics are given in Table 8.1.

We feel deep satisfaction at having increased national awareness on death and dying and having, day by day, demonstrated the efficiency of our services. The increase in the number of cases seen every year shows the positioning of Omega as a solid, ethically respectable professional entity that rises to the level of scientific societies.

**TABLE 8.1**

| Year | # Cases Assisted |
| --- | --- |
| 1986 | 0 |
| 1987 | 59 |
| 1988 | 101 |
| 1989 | 160 |
| 1990 | 242 |
| 1991 | 326 |
| 1992 | 526 |
| 1993 | 647 |
| 1994 | 782 |
| Total | 2,843 |

## WHAT WE STILL HAVE TO DO

Even though our balance sheet is highly satisfactory, there is still a long way to go. Demand for our services has increased, primarily because of favorable references given by a person or family who has benefited from Omega.

There is still not enough awareness of the need for these services in our country. In many cases, families come to us looking only for the handling of the agonies of the process, having deprived themselves of the possible benefit and enrichment that adequate and timely palliative care might have brought the family and the patient if sought in time.

Physicians, with rare exceptions, still do not send us patients. Paradoxically, as a proof of openness to new fields, they invite us more and more as lecturers in medical scientific events. These invitations come from the physicians who previously believed there was no need for this service for the dying patient, since they assumed that all the patient's needs could be met by them as professionals of medicine. They disregarded psychological and spiritual issues, and took care only of symptom control. They have now become convinced of the benefits of palliative care, especially when they have seen for themselves the benefits of specialized and holistic handling of the terminal phase of a patient in our hospice program.

We need still more academic space. Universities should open their doors to thanatology and palliative care . This would allow exposure of a larger number of physicians and nurses to more humanitarian care of dying patients.

Clinics and hospitals have been reluctant to accept palliative care because of a misconception that leads them to associate us with euthanasia. The need for palliative care also is not seen as a high priority.

In 1995, we begin to notice a change in this respect. We have begun conversations with heads of departments of oncology, and they are now contemplating the possibility of palliative care services within their own programs.

## WHAT ABOUT THE INPATIENT HOSPICE?

In 1992, we again became aware of the need for an inpatient unit, given the impossibility of the team's travelling to faraway homes.

We established enthusiastic and flexible contacts with private clinics. I found applause, but no effective support, in most cases. Two clinics finally considered the possibility, as a business matter, to make a partnership (nonprofit for Omega, of course) with Omega, and some insurance companies decided to support us because of my husband's connections and the presence of some insurance executives on our board.

During an entire year, we had "business" luncheons and conferences working towards a sensitization and motivation of the community towards the hospice project, again to be the first one in Colombia. We received 60% of the necessary budget—according to systematic and strenuous fact-finding studies—and not one more cent. I personally knocked on many doors and, sadly, they did not open. Once again, we had to return the donations we had already received and give up, until next time, our longed-for inpatient hospice unit. This unit remains necessary at this point of Omega's life for growth, for the establishment of a teaching unit on palliative care that would allow us to offer formal training to professionals. It would also enable us to have and to rely on well-paid team with research possibilities, this being an area that has been neglected because of lack of funding and available personnel.

## FOR THOSE WHO WISH TO BEGIN HOSPICE CARE

From our experience, we could offer six recommendations for those who might find themselves where we were in 1986.

1. Be ready for unforeseen situations and for a long, hard battle;
2. Evaluate the quality and solidity of the motivation of people who wish to join, so as to reduce desertion rates;
3. Designate a leader;
4. Do not stop training;
5. Establish limits for the professional activity of your institution, to exert an anchorlike function, flexibly allowing solidity and avoiding going adrift in the broad sea of promiscuity of alternatives that exist today. Be serious, but professional, and follow a line leading to your aim.
6. If possible, be politically, religiously, and academically independent.

## SOME UNFORGETTABLE LESSONS

As a member of a team that has learned, fought, cried, achieved, celebrated, and grown so much, I believe that there are thousands of daily lessons impossible to set on paper with reduced space.

On the personal level, each one of us has changed for the better. We have learned about the wealth of life, and also about the hidden wealth existing in the process of dying; we have learned that pain and problems do not mean weakness; we have learned to cry and accompany, and never to stop being moved by misfortune and suffering, but also to be able to do more with less suffering; and we have waive definitely learned to omnipotence, both as human beings and as professionals, and to humbly recognize that in many cases all we can offer is our presence.

Each one of the 13 team members daily expresses their gratitude towards the teachers who broadened our horizons; towards our beloved, those relatives and patients we loved and who lit our way with their deaths; towards our families, unending sources of faith, support, and patience; and towards life that gave us, like privileged beings, this beautiful chance to live with and for a better dying.

# 9

# Hospice Care in the United States

## Robert Kastenbaum

---

*Number of hospice programs in the United States:*
1973: 0          Today: 2000+

The rapid development of hospice care programs in the United States is best understood within the sociomedical context of its origins. This context has not remained fixed in time, no more than the challenges and opportunities faced by the hospice movement. It will be useful, then, to describe hospice care in the United States as it was, as it is, and as it may yet become.

## THE EMERGENCE OF HOSPICE CARE IN THE UNITED STATES

Few people had cancer and almost nobody died. This remarkable fact was shadowed by another fact that one was not supposed to notice—nearly half a million "passed away" each year after a "lingering illness." "Cancer," "death," and "dying" were words not to be spoken in polite society nor, for that matter, in the classrooms where future human service professionals were learning the rudiments of their craft. The development of hospice care programs would not have been possible without a major attitudinal shift on the part of both the general public and human service professionals. Several of the factors that contributed to this shift will be explored here, though quite briefly.

## Health Care in the American Death System: 1960s–1970s

The modern version of hospice care was taking shape in the 1960s, primarily in the United Kingdom, under the leadership of Cicely Saunders. In the United States, there were individual nurses, physicians, clergypersons, and social scientists who were concerned about the ordeals frequently experienced by dying persons, but there were as yet no fully realized palliative care programs.

It has been observed that every society has a "death system," i.e., a network of symbols and action tendencies that mediate the individual's relationship with mortality (Kastenbaum, 1995). The major functions of a death system are warning and prediction, prevention, caring for the dying, disposing of the dead, social consolidation after death, making sense of death, and the regulation of killing. The relative priority of these functions can differ from society to society, and is subject to change within the same society. By the 1960s, the American health care system had sharply increased the priority of the warning-prediction-prevention (cure) orientation. As this end of the seesaw continued to rise, there was a corresponding decline in attention given to caring for the dying person, disposing of the dead, and social consolidation following the death. The meaning of death had become an almost irrelevant question within the health care system.

It was not simply that the health care system was more interested in prevention and cures than in caring for the terminally ill. The imbalance had become excessive and pervasive. If, for example, we "follow the money," it is evident that funding for research and technological development was poured into the prevention/cure endeavor, with less than token support for supportive and palliative care. Moreover, the incentives for a brilliant and prosperous career were almost totally concentrated in prevention/cure. The idea of preparing medical students to help terminally ill people achieve a "good death" was definitely out of fashion.

The aggressive war against death that characterized the leading edge of the American health care system by the 1960s also turned away from the ever-growing population of elders. For example, there was stiff resistance to the suggestion that a specialty be created in geriatric medicine. A practice with nursing home residents and other elders was considered to be near the bottom of the barrel. Those care providers and scientists who pioneered the emerging field of gerontology at this time did so with the realization that their colleagues tended to consider this activity as useless, depressing, and lacking in prestige.

"Real" medicine was the enthusiastic application of the new diagnostic and treatment modalities provided by science and technology. The preference was for "interesting" patients. One became an interesting patient through being a viable candidate for the latest procedures that fascinated and enriched hospital systems and physicians. Terminally ill and aged patients would attract attention so long as they provided the opportunity for medical learning experiences. When perceived as merely dying or old, however, they would either be ejected from the prime health care system, into the burgeoning long-term care facilities, or isolated within the hospital, with minimal care. Many dying persons and many elders with multiple age-related conditions felt rejected. They *were* rejected.

This technologically enhanced, cure-driven orientation rapidly changed the preexisting health care system and its relationship with the public. The new medicine, though, had to compete with expectations that had established themselves in the public mind over many decades. One of the most important of these expectations was for a personal relationship with a physician who would provide care in his/her office and in the patient's home. Most people were "dead set" against entering a hospital. This attitude was especially strong among mid-life and elderly adults, who often had personal and family memories of negative hospital experiences. As Rosenberg (1995) has documented, the reputation of hospitals had become tainted, first by their early character as public welfare institutions with appalling conditions, and then by their professionalized but increasingly impersonal and bureaucratic orientation toward the patient.

Now the hospital had become a place where many people were treated successfully for acute conditions—a positive development that nevertheless did not extend to sensitive care for the chronically and terminally ill. The dying person did not quite fit into the philosophy and practice of the new-style hospital; this person was likely to be "acute" with respect to symptom management, but "chronic" in the sense that the condition was not amenable to remission over time. In essence, the dying person did not fit into the increasingly dominant techno-bureaucratic health care system.

## Attitudes Toward Death and Dying

The hospital system was not the only sphere in which the dying person had little visibility or priority. As already noted, even such words as "cancer," "dying," and "death" were avoided in the classroom, the media, and personal conversation. At the surface level, it appeared that people were attempting to spare each other the anxieties aroused by the acknowledgement of death. It was considered cruel and tactless to speak directly of death, especially to people who were anticipating or had experienced a loss. Nevertheless, it was not difficult to observe that the considerate people who were avoiding the subject of death were also attempting to control their own anxieties. This phenomenon is commonly reported by adults who recall their childhood experiences during the 1950s through the 70s (Kastenbaum, 1995). With few exceptions, they report that their parents maintained an anxious and avoidant silence about death. "It was something you could never talk or ask about!" is a typical memory. When these "children of the taboo" became parents, they found it difficult to respond helpfully to their children's questions and experiences.

As might be expected within this attitudinal context, there was also a prevailing fear and reluctance to interact directly with dying people and their family members (both before and after the death). Many a tragicocomic situation arose in which friends, colleagues, and neighbors awkwardly attempted to console a grieving person without exactly mentioning the nature of the loss and without exactly being ready to listen to what the survivor might be impelled to say. Indeed, *communication apprehension* was a salient feature of death-related interactions in the U.S. Teachers and clergymen, as well as the person next door, often felt surges of anxiety at the prospect of having to interact with a person who had been touched by death in some way. Professionals could try to conceal their own uneasiness by relying on cliches and generalizations, but would often betray their anxiety through nonverbal ("body") language and the inclination to "split the scene" as soon as possible. The care process—like all interpersonal transactions—relies on effective mutual communication. For many years, death-related communications were effective chiefly in reducing the length, scope, accuracy, and intimacy of interactions with dying and grieving people.

Curiously—or, perhaps, not so curiously—the public allowed itself to be titillated by violent death. The emergence of television as the dominant medium provided the opportunity for the even more extensive proliferation of shoot-'em-up and explode-those-crashing-cars programming. Both factual and fictional violence attracted the attentional energies of a public that could not deal with "natural" death in real life. Gorer's (1965) analysis of "the pornography of death" seemed to apply to the U.S. as well as his native England: there may be a parallel between the increased interest in reports of "kinky" or "abnormal" sex and death along with a decreased ability to cope with "natural" sex and death. Gorer did not believe censorship to be the right approach to pornographic sex and death. Instead, he asserted that "People have to come to terms with the basic facts of birth, copulation, and death, and somehow accept their implications; if social prudery prevents this being done in an open and dignified fashion, then it will be done surreptitiously. . . . If we make death unmentionable in polite society—'not before the children'—we almost ensure the continuation of the 'horror comic'." (p. 217)

Gorer's call for the restoration of "natural death" to public discourse was soon to be heeded.

## Hospice Care Enters the Scene

The first "official" hospice in the United States made its appearance in 1974. Hospice, Inc. (New Haven, Connecticut) was founded only seven years after Cicely Saunders established St. Christopher's Hospice in England, which almost immediately became the beacon and model for hospice programs worldwide. The connection was close in personnel and concept as well as in time. The first medical director of Hospice, Inc. was Sylvia Lack, who had served as a physician with St. Christopher's and had first-hand experience with Saunders' ideals and techniques. Florence Wald and Ed Dobihal acquired knowledge of hospice philosophy and practice in sabbaticals at St. Christopher's and were also able to bring this experience to the Connecticut venture. As subsequent history reveals, this program took root after a period of struggle, and soon the hospice spirit was expressing itself in other nascent efforts throughout the nation.

How was it possible for hospice care to take root in the U. S. so quickly? Two major sources of influence should be noted, although other forces were also at work.

Consumerism and the "Return-to-Nature" movement may be taken as two facets of the same trend. Americans wanted to gain or regain control of their lives. Ralph Nader and other activists demonstrated that it was possible for the "passive consumer" to exercise influence over major corporations. It was a long way from pressuring automakers to increase the safety of their products to creating an alternative to traditional care of the dying person. Nevertheless, public success in criticizing even the most powerful strongholds of the establishment carried over into the realm of personal health and quality of life. The return-to-nature movement expressed itself through a revival of interest in organic foods and drugs, exercise, and whatever pursuits seemed to promise an escape from the manufactured and mass-mediated world (although, of course, the nature movement generated its own products and rhetoric). "Natural birth" became a particularly influential rallying call. "Natural death" soon followed as a natural correlate.

The other major source of influence was the death awareness movement (referred to by some as *thanatology*). This movement had both popular and professional/academic components. Two more British imports captured the fancy of the American reading public. Evelyn Waugh's (1948) gentle send-up of Forest Lawn-type funeral practices in *The Loved One* made a delayed impact after the success of Jessica Mitford's (1963) caustic observations on the funeral industry, *The American Way of Death*. These were relatively safe death topics for the public. One could have some laughs at the expense of the funeral industry without having one's most personal anxieties pricked. Discourse about death was now possible within the limited realm of "those foolish" or "knavish" funeral directors (almost needless to say, both books presented caricatures, rather than balanced portraits of the American funeral process).

A scattering of researchers and professional caregivers was also starting to turn its attention to death-related issues. Whether psychiatrists, psychologists, nurses, sociologists, anthropologists, social workers, or clergy, these people tended to work alone at first. There would be the local "grief lady" who could be counted on to listen to a family's sorrows, or the researcher who unaccountably was wasting time on death and dying when everybody else was engaged with more rewarding topics. Several breakthrough works finally drew some attention to death-related topics on the part of the professional services and research communities. Herman Feifel's (1959) edited book, *The Meaning of Death* was the first of the new wave to take hold, and it anticipated future trends by including contributions from various disciplines. Other books and articles followed, many of which focused on the social isolation of the dying person. *Omega,* the first professional/scientific journal devoted to death-related topics, published its first issue in 1970, providing a much-needed information channel for the newly emerging field of death studies.

The first courses on death were also introduced during this period (the middle 60s and early 70s), along with public lectures and workshops. "Death education" became so popular for a while that it did not entirely escape the criticism of being a "fad," but there was both substance and passion as well. Observations made by a growing number of researchers were documenting the human needs of the dying person, just as the public was finding its voice to protest what was perceived as cold and impersonal treatment on the part of the health care establishment. A number of practitioners within the health care system joined wholeheartedly into the crusade. The most influential of these insiders was Elizabeth Kubler-Ross, whose (1969) book, *On Death and Dying,* and lecture tours struck a particularly responsive chord.

Whether coincidence or not, the early peak of interest in death education occurred in the brief interval between founding of London's St. Christopher's Hospice and New Haven's Hospice, Inc. There was now an aroused public with a willingness to "speak about the unspeakable" and explore new avenues for improving the quality of life—including life in the shadow of death.

## Money and Mercy: Crossing the Feasibility Threshold

Despite an improved social climate for improving terminal care, the hospice movement faced major obstacles. There was a major educational task ahead. Both care providers and the public would have to understand what hospice was and what it was not. Long-entrenched patterns of behavior would have to be altered, including the premises involved in communicational interactions between professional caregivers and patients/families. Looming above the other challenges, however, was the availability of funding. Who would pay for hospice care?

The complete story of hospice's struggle for financial support has yet to be told. It is a remarkable story, considering that the threshold of hospice survival was crossed during the Reagan administration, whose policies were not favorable to social programs, especially the innovative. In one of history's many ironic twists, it was the cost-cutting mission of the Reagan administration that contributed mightily to hospice gaining its toe-hold. The Health Care Finance Administration

(HCFA) decided it was worth the risk to invest in a demonstration project that would give hospice programs the opportunity to show what they could do. An evaluation component was included. The support was temporary and contingent: if hospice did not do in practice what it advocated in theory, then the experiment was over. Hospice had to do more than provide competent care, however. It had to save money. Both the grassroots and the professional/research constituents of the death awareness movement were gratified by the federal response, yet the decision was to be made primarily on the basis of money, not mercy.

Results from the largest study of the demonstration project (Mor, 1987; Mor, Greer, & Kastenbaum, 1988) did not favor hospice care in a clear across-the-board comparison with hospital care. (One of the major difficulties here was the continuing difficulty in obtaining reliable, consistent, and meaningful measures of pain.) Nevertheless, the general pattern was encouraging. Hospice programs did what they said they would do (e.g., utilize fewer expensive and invasive medical procedures), and some key findings did emerge (e.g., more days spent at home). HCFA decided that hospice programs could help to control the medical expenses of the terminal phase of life while providing an acceptable level of care. Many families as well as hospice staff and volunteers were firm in their opinion that hospice care was more than an acceptable alternative: "It was a godsend!" reported a woman whose husband had been one of the first hospice patients.

Hospice became an option to Medicaid-funded hospitalization in 1982. The emphasis was on home care. The typical hospice patient was a man or woman over the age of 60 with some form of terminal cancer. People who knew about hospice could make an informed choice, assuming the availability of a hospice program in their community. There was now a foundation of economic support for hospice programs (along with a set of certification requirements and regulations). Nevertheless, few hospices could function adequately on the basis of federal reimbursements alone. Hospices would have to find ways to develop additional funding sources if they were to meet the needs of their communities. Therefore, many hospice programs turned—and still turn—to their local communities for financial support. Mercy still needs money.

## HOSPICE TODAY

After two decades, hospice care has itself become part of the health system establishment that it once challenged. Actually, the challenge continues, and it goes both ways. Hospice programs deserve credit for improvements that can be observed in some hospital settings. Physicians and nurses who have learned hospice philosophy and techniques are bringing their enhanced skills into the hospital setting. Meanwhile, hospital systems have themselves launched hospice programs. These programs tend to differ in subtle, and not always subtle, ways from the first set of hospice programs that were created during the earlier mission-driven years. With the best of intentions, hospital administrators (and their boards of directors) have a frame of reference and expectation that differs from the vision of those who strove to introduce the hospice concept with a sense of urgency and passion. In the larger picture, the situation is as described by Corless (1995):

> The price of becoming a part of the system was to lose the charismatic elements of a social movement and become tamed, albeit legitimized by the system. The hospice movement was co-opted by the federal establishment. The cost of such bureacratization was to limit access to hospice to those who might have been sustained at home by traditional home-care agencies (p. 79).

As Corless also suggests, the cost of legitimization has included the need to focus time and energy on compliance with regulatory agencies and being pressured to make decisions on the basis of reimbursement opportunities. It is not easy to keep the sense of mission alive when hospice directors are saddled with fiscal and management responsibilities that are peripheral to the actual care of terminally ill people and their families.

Despite such problems, hospice care has exercised a continuing positive influence, not only in the terminal care situation, but also in its demonstration that people can come together to offer support for each other during life's challenges and ordeals. The pessimism and frustration often experienced within the cauldron of mass society is countered every time hospice volunteers and staff show anew that people have the power to help people.

These demonstrations of help occur more than 200,000 times a year in the U.S.A. (Beresford, 1993, p. 9). More than four out of five hospice patients have cancer, and about one in every three who die of cancer has selected the hospice option. To be eligible for the hospice option, Americans must be certified by a physician as having 6 months or less to live. This is often a difficult and unwelcome task for the physician. The tendency is to delay issuing this certification as long as possible—and then, perhaps, a little longer. Along with the reluctance to err by making a premature judgment of terminality, physicians are often reluctant to turn management of a patient over to hospice until the last moment. As a result, it is not uncommon for hospices to meet their patients only a few weeks—or days—before death. This can hardly be considered the optimal use of hospice skills, nor the most compassionate service to the patient. Even without this problematic length-of-life requirement, it is a challenge in each case to determine the optimal point for transition from cure-oriented to comfort-oriented care.

Several types of hospice organizations operate in the U.S. Beresford (1993) characterizes these models as follows:

- *Community-based:* Independent, nonprofit corporations. Advantage: caring for the dying is its only mission. Disadvantage: financial instability, because it is not part of a larger organization.
- *Home health agency-based:* A unit within a visiting nurse association or public health nursing department. Advantage: part of a home-care oriented agency. Disadvantage: lacks the full range and intensiveness of hospice services.
- *Hospital-based:* A unit of a hospital corporation. Advantage: can draw upon the personnel and other resources of the parent organization. Disadvantage: "the needs of a small hospice department sometimes get lost in a large institution that places too much emphasis on the bottom line" (p. 78).
- *Volunteer-intensive:* Small agencies operating in isolated rural areas; usually belong to a larger unit (any of the above), but depend almost entirely on unpaid staff. Advantage: sense of mission and neighborliness. Disadvantage: limited resources available.
- *Freestanding:* Operates its own physical facilities within the community. Advantage: more control over decision-making. Disadvantage: less cost-effective, so more vulnerable to financial problems.

There are subtypes within some of these models, as well as hybrid hospice organizations that include the characteristics of two or more models.

Another differentiation has also appeared on the U.S. hospice scene: *proprietary*, as distinguished from *nonprofit*. For some time, virtually all U.S. hospices operated on a nonprofit basis. Scattered attempts were made to establish profitmaking hospices, but few, if any, took root. Today, there are a number of proprietary hospices in operation. These tend to be franchise enterprises controlled by large national corporations. Beresford (1993) observes that:

> To some in the American hospice care movement, a proprietary hospice seems somehow contrary to hospice's idealistic tradition, as does the aggressive marketing of hospice services. However, there is no evidence that proprietary hospices are less expert or dedicated in the care they provide, or that their services are less satisfactory to patients and families (p. 80).

It should be noted that most people do not actually have a choice between these various models. There may be only one type of hospice care organization available in a community.

Palliative care services for children are receiving more attention than in the past, most often through enhanced home-care programs. As Corr & Corr (1993, p. 142) note:

> The structure or location of the program is less important than its holistic approach and its effectiveness in serving the needs of each child-and-family unit.

## HOSPICE TOMORROW

The shape, scope, and even the survival of hospice programs in the U.S. depend upon many biosocial forces and the judgment of its decisionmakers. Here are some of the challenges with which hospice must cope to follow its path into the future.

### Access for Patients Without Live-in Primary Caregivers

As already noted, strict enforcement of regulations would deprive many people of hospice care (e.g., an elderly person who lives alone). Action is now being taken to test the feasibility of hospice care for people who are now excluded for lack of a live-in caregiver, and the early results are encouraging (Bly & Kissick, 1994).

### Access for Members of Ethnic and Racial Minorities

Stoddard (1990) is among those who have pointed out that the hospice movement has not encompassed all segments of society to an equal degree. This assessment remains true today. There is little basis for accusing hospice leaders of deliberately excluding particular populations, but circumstances have nevertheless contributed to this outcome. A major challenge here is the encouragement of hospice activism within subgroups who seldom have the opportunity to utilize palliative services. The needs of terminally ill people must compete with many other urgent needs in these populations.

### Coping with Terminal-Phase AIDS Patients

This challenge already exists for most hospices. Some public health officials project a significant increase in terminal-phase AIDS in the years ahead; others believe the magnitude has been somewhat overestimated. Whatever the numbers, the emergence of AIDS is presenting new problems in symptom management and contagion control for caregivers. Furthermore, hospice staff, volunteers, and fundraisers must deal with public uneasiness regarding a medical condition that is still stigmatized and still not fully understood. The future may hold other unexpected challenges from diseases that are today obscure or unknown, as well as from the possible casualties of diseases that have learned how to overcome antibiotic treatment.

### Providing Effective Care for Patients with a Broader Spectrum of Terminal Conditions

Heart disease in its various forms remains the most common cause of death in the U.S. Nevertheless, relatively few people with high cardiac risk avail themselves of palliative care services. As already noted, hospice care has been to a large extent the care of people with end-phase cancer. It also appears particularly well suited to the care of elderly individuals, in a society that is growing older all the time (Levy, 1994). Whether or not the hospice philosophy can be applied extensively to people suffering from a much broader spectrum of conditions remains to be seen.

## Will Volunteers Continue to Be Available in Sufficient Numbers?

It is difficult to imagine hospice care programs without a complement of dedicated and skillful volunteers. Attrition occurs as volunteers move away or find it necessary to give their attention to other interests and obligations. Furthermore, it has been found that some volunteers quit because of anxieties directly related to their hospice experiences (Lafer, 1991). Attrition need not be a threat to hospice survival as long as the rate is low or moderate and a fresh supply of volunteers can be recruited. It is possible, though, that the "two-paycheck family" will seriously reduce the number of qualified hospice volunteers as people find it necessary to devote more time to remunerated work. Whatever other forces reduce the pool or increase the competition for volunteers could place hospice volunteer programs in jeopardy.

## Will the Spiritual Dimensions of Care Continue to Flourish in a Technological, Materialistic, and Competitive Society?

The concepts of spiritual pain and spiritual care have been with hospice since the start, and have been reaffirmed by Saunders, Baines, and Dunlop (1995) and Wald (1986). Research has found that almost all volunteers report themselves to be people with a sense of spiritual mission and engage frequently in prayer for guidance and strength (Schneider & Kastenbaum, 1993). The hardiness of the spiritual approach has been proven through the centuries, but emerging pressures, stresses, and distractions should not be underestimated. Still untested is the possibility that hospice care could retain its compassionate and holistic approach without a core of spirituality.

## Is Assisted Suicide a Threat to Hospice Care?

Academic debates about a "right to die" have already been eclipsed by events. In the U.S., Jack Kevorkian, M.D., has been reported as assisting in the deaths of 35 people (some of whom were not terminally ill). Courts, legislative bodies, and care providers are grappling with the assisted death issue while public controversy swirls. How this drama will continue to play out remains to be seen. The implications for hospice care programs are also unclear. For example, Logue

(1994) has discussed "the limits of palliative care" and suggested that a point may come for some patients in which assisted death could be considered a realistic and ethical option. Saunders (1995–96) has countered with an articulation and defense of hospice principles. There will be many more such differences of opinion as public opinion, professional practice, and judicial/legal decisionmaking interact around this emotional and consequential issue. The question of how hospice programs should address the assisted death issue is not without implications for the future of hospice care.

Whatever the future may bring to the health care system in the U.S., one may hope that it will include a vigorous, resilient, and effective palliative care component.

## REFERENCES

Beresford, L. (1993). *The hospice handbook.* Boston: Little, Brown.

Bly, J. L., & Kissick, P. (1994). Hospice care for patients living alone: Results of a demonstration program. *The Hospice Journal, 9,* 9–20.

Corless, I. B. (1995). A new decade for hospice. In I. B. Corless, B. B. Germino, & M. A. Pittman (Eds.), *A challenge for living* (pp. 77–94). Boston: Jones & Bartlett.

Corr, C. A., & Corr, D. M. (1993). Hospice: Children. In R. Kastenbaum & B. K. Kastenbaum (Eds.), *The Encyclopedia of Death* (pp. 141–143). Phoenix: Oryx Press.

Feifel, H. (Ed.) (1959). *The meaning of death.* New York: McGraw-Hill.

Gallagher-Allred, C., & Amenta, M. O'R. (Eds.) (1993). Nutrition and hydration in hospice care: Needs, strategies, ethics [special issue]. *The Hospice Journal, 9* (2–3).

Gorer, G. (1965). The pornography of death. In G. Gorer (Ed.), *Death, grief, and mourning* (pp. 210–221). New York: Doubleday.

Kastenbaum, R. (1995). *Death, society, and human experience* (5th ed.). Boston: Allyn & Bacon.

Kübler-Ross, E. (1969). *On death and dying.* New York: Macmillan.

Lafer, B. (1991). The attrition of hospice volunteers. *Omega: Journal of Death and Dying, 23,* 161–168.

Levy, J. A. (1994). The hospice in the context of an aging society. In R. Fulton & R. Bendikson (Eds.), *Death and identity* (3rd ed.) (pp. 364–381). Philadelphia: Charles Press.

Logue, B. J. (1994). When hospice fails: The limits of palliative care. *Omega: Journal of Death and Dying, 29,* 291–302.

Logue, B. J. (1995–1996). Rejoinder to Saunders. *Omega: Journal of Death and Dying, 32,* 7–9.

Mitford, J. (1963). *The American way of death.* New York: Simon & Schuster.

Mor, V. (1987). *Hospice care systems.* New York: Springer Publishing Co.

Mor, V., Greer, D. S., & Kastenbaum, R. (Eds.) (1988). *The hospice experiment.* Baltimore: The Johns Hopkins University Press.

Rosenberg, C. E. (1995). *The care of strangers.* Baltimore: The Johns Hopkins University Press.

Saunders, C. 1995–1996, 32, 7–10. A response to Logue's "Where hospice fails: The limits of palliative care." *Omega: Journal of Death and Dying, 32,* 1–6.

Saunders, C., Baines, M., & Dunlop, R. (1995). *Living with dying: A guide to palliative care* (3rd ed.). Oxford: Oxford University Press.

Schneider, S., & Kastenbaum, R. (1993). Patterns and meanings of prayer in hospice caregivers. *Death Studies, 17,* 471–485.

Stoddard, S. (1990). Hospice: Approaching the 21st century. *The American Journal of Hospice and Palliative Care, 7,* 27–30.

Wald, F. (Ed.) (1986). *In quest of the spiritual component of care for the terminally ill.* New Haven: Yale University Press.

Wald, F. (1994). Finding a way to give hospice care: A nurse's diary. In I. B. Corless, B. B. Germino, & M. Pittman (Eds.), *Dying, death, and bereavement* (pp. 31–47). Boston: Jones & Bartlett.

Waugh, E. (1948). *The loved one.* Boston: Little, Brown.

# *Australasia*

# 10

# Hawke's Bay: A New Zealand Approach to Hospice Care

## Dr. Malcolm Joblin and Staff, Cranford Hospice

---

*Sarah very quickly became much weaker. Although she had wanted to walk into the Hospice, she had to go by ambulance when the time came. The ambulance pulled up at the Hospice verandah where a nurse met Sarah with a wheelchair. As she was wheeled along the verandah, Sarah was thrilled to see the wisteria running the full length, great billowing bouquets of pale purple cascading all around her. She was soon sipping a cup of tea and already beginning to relax in the peace and quiet of the Hospice, a big old villa similar to the house in which she had grown up. Sarah had felt so uncomfortable before she came to the Hospice that she thought that this was probably her last effort, and that she would die there in a matter of days. Instead, 3 days later, she walked out, leaning only lightly on the arm of the same nurse who had wheeled her in. Sarah went home with her daughter. The Hospice home support nurse visited them at home daily. Her family drew up an informal roster so that there was always someone with her when she needed them. Twelve days later, Sarah died peacefully in her own bed.*

*Bill felt that he now had enough strength to take himself for a short walk through the Hospice grounds. He tucked the newspaper under his arm, waved to the nurse, and stepped slowly out the door. Ever since he had arrived at the Hospice he had wanted to check out the vegetable garden, and now he saw that the climbing beans were a riot of*

*red flowers, just as the garderner had said. The rhubarb was enormous. There was a*
*forest of silver beet and masses of mint and parsley. Now he walked over to the gazebo,*
*sat down gently with just a twinge of pain in his thigh, and unfurled the paper.*

*He thought that he had better tell them that there was still a bit of pain after all. Then*
*he remembered what it had been like before he came to the Hospice. That set his mind*
*to recalling how it had been when his wife died. It had not been long ago really, but there*
*was no Hospice then. She was in a hospital. The pain was awful. The hospital staff was*
*wonderful, but Bill knew that palliative medicine was in its infancy at that time and was*
*not taught in either the medical schools or the nursing schools. They used to give her what*
*was called a Brompton's cocktail, which he knew contained morphine, cocaine, and*
*chlorpromazine. When his wife could talk, she said she felt terrible. Later, when she*
*couldn't swallow, they gave her intramuscular injections of morphine. These were*
*provided only on a strict schedule, and she would groan in pain several hours before the*
*next dose was due. She also had chlorpromazine injections, but looked frightened and*
*miserable for much of the time.*

*Bill also remembered that there was no single room available for his wife and*
*the nurses were always very busy. He decided he wouldn't think about that any more.*

## THE FOUNDING OF CRANFORD HOSPICE

Cranford Hospice was founded in 1982. Before that time, people with terminal
illnesses were managed in medical or surgical wards in hospitals, or at home with
whatever support could be arranged. There was no coordinated terminal care and
palliative medicine was not a recognized entity. There were only three other
hospices in the whole of New Zealand.

Jack Mackie was the Chief Executive Officer of the local Presbyterian Support
Services (PSS) organization, a church-based community agency whose activities
included homes and hospitals for elderly people and family assistance programs.
He and his wife listened to their daughter's expressions of frustration as a hospital
nurse who was unable to spend time with dying patients. They agreed that there
had to be a better way.

On a subsequent overseas trip, the Mackies made a point of visiting hospices
and found that, indeed, there was a better way. They come home with the dream
of starting a palliative care program in Hawke's Bay. Thus began the slow, time-
consuming, and often frustrating process of bringing the dream to fruition. The
PSS Board entered the dream when they agreed to purchase a large house that had
become available after it was no longer needed to serve as a geriatric hospital. This
building was to become a hospice to serve Hawke's Bay, a province that include
two small cities with a catchment area of more than 120,000 people.

Hours were spent talking to community organizations, outlining what was in
mind, and gaining their assistance. A committee was set up, comprised of an

Anglican priest who was jointly employed at that time by PSS and Anglican Social Services; a nurse who was then deputy principal of one of the PASS geriatric home/hospitals; and a hospital pharmacist who had recently returned from Volunteer Service Abroad. A former member of Parliament was employed to speak to local groups and enlist their support.

Every community group they could identify was contacted and involved in the project. Businesses were approached for financial and practical help (e. g., supplying furnishings and other materials). By the beginning of 1982, the rooms had been carpeted by several local firms. All the rooms had been wallpapered, and equipment was in place. Most of the work was done by volunteers. Local people gave generously of their time, service, and money. The most active responders were women's groups, such as the Country Women's Institutes and church organizations.

Committee members visited one of the three hospices that had been identified as most similar to the vision they had in mind of a small, short-stay community hospice. The same committee interviewed prospective staff, both professional and ancillary. When the Hospice became operational later that year, most of its staff were volunteers.

Medical care was first provided by the patient's family doctor. This was not always an ideal arrangement, however, as few had had any training in palliative medicine. Furthermore, with the wide cachement area of the Hospice, many doctors were not close enough to provide the immediate care needed. In time, a medical director was appointed. There was some resistance to this appointment from local general practitioners and specialists. This resistance was probably occasioned by a sense of having been excluded to some extent, or perhaps because they were unable to recognize at the time that the Hospice was providing, or indeed was capable of providing, a specialized service.

For some community physicians, the problem was that the medical director was a woman. A hint of this resistance persists at times even today, but on the whole it has been overwhelmed by recognition of the excellent service that is provided by the Hospice program.

## CRANFORD HOSPICE TODAY

Although founded and operated under the auspices of a Presbyterian church organization, Cranford Hospice is nondenominational and nonreligious. There are only six beds, but at times as many as one hundred people are listed as patients and are at home. Some of these patients are still undergoing active treatment, such as chemotherapy, through one of the local hospitals, or radiotherapy at the regional oncology service, which is two hours away by road.

We offer relief and comfort to people with a terminal illness and to those looking after them. The Hospice also acts as a resource center for those involved in palliative care. The aims of the Hospice are to meet the physical, emotional, and spiritual needs of the patients and their families. Most people come to Cranford for only a few days, and then return to their homes. Some return several times. Most people come to find relief from pain, anxiety, or other symptoms, such as nausea and vomiting. Some patients come primarily so that their caregivers can have a much needed rest. Others come seeking expert care in the final stages of their illness.

Patients often are referred by their family doctor or specialist. The referral can also be at their own request. A team of nurses, doctors, pharmacist and a chaplain is available day and night every day of the year. The 24-hour Hospice telephone is staffed by nurses to provide advice, support, and reassurance both to patients and their families. Hospice support nurses visit people in their homes 7 days a week, offering practical assistance, comfort, and advice, as well as communicating with family doctors, community health services, and Hospice staff.

A two-bedroom flat is attached to the Hospice and is available to family and friends of patients.

Most patients have cancer, but there are no exclusion criteria.

The service is available free of charge to everyone regardless of age, race, beliefs, or financial situation.

Bereavement followup is provided by a team of volunteers, and ongoing support is available. Other volunteers provide cleaning, cooking, gardening, laundry, fundraising, and the many other essential activities of day-to-day running of the establishment, without which it would cease to function.

There is a paid volunteer coordinator who organizes this small army of helpers. Paid and volunteer office staff help keep things running. The Principal Nurse/Manager is in charge on-site. The Chief Executive Officer of the PSS and the PSS Board manage affairs on a larger scale.

No patient is expected to pay for any Hospice service. Until 1994, there was no direct financial input from central government. Since then, a contract with a governmental health funding agency has ensured funding for 50% of Cranford's expenditure. Nevertheless, we are still heavily dependent on income from legacies and bequests, grants from charitable trusts, and donations from local businesses and the community we serve.

One of the more spectacular fundraising ventures is a charity wine auction, the culmination of a weekend of activity during a national holiday. Many of the local wineries for which the region is famous donate bottles and barrels of their wine. After tastings and banquets and often much hilarity, the wine is auctioned for both ridiculously low and amazingly high prices and the proceeds given to Cranford Hospice. This weekend has now become an institution, and in its most recent manifestation raised more than $80,000 from the auction alone.

After 14 years of operation, Cranford Hospice is well-established. There is always more to learn, so that ongoing education is essential. Regular attendances at conferences, interchange between hospices, tutorials for all staff (for instance, by local and visiting specialists), and other training programs ensure that we keep up to date. We aim to be open to new practices, and are careful not to use only those methods which we have found effective in the past.

There is little audit of any health practices in New Zealand, but we must be open to scrutiny and prepared to participate in assessment programs. We must, and indeed we do, teach others what we know. Our staff provide on-the-job tuition for personnel from nearby hospices, thereby ensuring that our sort of care is more widely available.

## CHALLENGES

We still face many challenges. Funding will probably always be one of these challenges. We must continue to try to impress upon the government that palliative care, like all other aspects of health, needs to be properly funded.

To some extent, we have been our own worst enemy by providing an essential service in an efficient manner with resources supplied, until recently, by the community. The government has felt little need to spend any of its tax money on the care of the terminally ill. We also need to keep the work of hospice in the minds of the people, maintaining community interest in our activities so the public will continue to donate, bequeath, and fundraise for our cause. More and more the public is having to dip into its pockets for other causes, so at times it can be a struggle to compete for available dollars.

Another challenge is that of recognition by some allied professionals that we are providing a specialized service and that indeed we are working *with* them, rather than in opposition to them. Meeting this challenge is mostly a matter of communication—and communication we know to be vital, especially in our line of work.

To some extent—and, fortunately, to a diminishing extent—there is still a public misapprehension that a hospice is a place to which you go to die, and only when you are just about to die. This belief often becomes a self-fulfilling prophecy. This, too, is a challenge to us. *We continue to impress upon everyone that we want to become involved in the care of people as early as possible in their illness, so that they can live well until they die.* Some of the misapprehension has its roots in fear, especially the fear of dying. We must continue to allay this fear. Our cause is not helped by death notices in the newspaper which announce that the person died "at Cranford Hospice." Although it is probably good to keep our name in people's minds, it is a sort of negative publicity which keeps afloat the myth that hospices are places where people die. We still need to explain our role and the benefits of early association with our service. There are still people to be reached.

People seldom associate hospices with fun, but laughter is often heard emanating from our rooms. Staff members are neither morbid nor overly consumed with death. We all like a good laugh and have had some hilarious experiences at work. This aspect of hospice life is often overlooked, but it is essential to the emotional strength and sanity of us all.

Hospice people need to work as a team, and many of our important decisions are made only after team meetings in which all views are aired. We do have the odd argument, but acrimony doesn't last long in our environment. And we do have to be careful that making a team decision does not mean making policies about a particular aspect of management that contravene someone else's codes of practice.

The hospice movement in New Zealand is still a relatively new one. Early hospices such as ours were instrumental in founding umbrella organizations, such as Hospice New Zealand, which are now establishing guidelines and suggestions for good palliative care. There are now many hospices throughout the country offering a wide range of services of various magnitudes.

We recognize the importance of communication so that we don't all have to reinvent the wheel. Experiences and problems—especially those confronted in trying to get a new hospice up and running—need to be shared freely. At times, a spirit of competition and rivalry has sneaked into contact between Hospices. This negativistic spirit has no place in effective palliative care, and should be exorcised whenever detected.

We should be able to guarantee to our patient, Bill, all the things his wife could not expect only a few years ago: dignity, excellent symptom control, and dedicated care at all levels, from early in the illness right through to a peaceful end.

*Europe*

# 11

# Palliative Medicine's First Steps in Croatia

Anica Jusic

---

## VISITING ST. CHRISTOPHER'S HOSPICE

Before retirement I worked as a clinical neurologist, dealing especially with neuromuscular diseases. I founded and lead a center for neuromuscular diseases in Zagreb, and had taught neurology and electromyography as a university professor for more than 30 years, organizing symposia, workshops, and courses.

My special concern was for patients suffering and dying with devastating motor neurone disease (Amyotropic Lateral sclerosis, also known as Lou Gehrig's Disease). It was difficult to help them. There was not even a consensus that it was worthwhile to try to manage the signs and symptoms of fatal motor neurone disease, or on what patterns of symptomatic treatment might be useful. I was, therefore, quite interested in participating in The First International Symposium on Amyotrophic Lateral Sclerosis/Motor Neurone Disease, held in Solihull, England in 1990. One evening during dinner in Birmingham, I was told that physicians sent their problem patients to St. Christopher's Hospice. It was then that I first heard about Dame Cicely Saunders and the hospice movement. I asked a friend in Wimbledon if she could arrange for me to have a short visit at St. Christopher's. The few hours I spent there with my friend determined my future occupation.

St. Christopher's made a strong impression on me. This impression began when I noticed the wide hospice entrance with simple, functional furniture, flowers, pictures on the walls, and small children running about. The impression continued to grow as we were met by Dame Cicely Saunders, who accepted us warmly, as if we were old friends. Throughout the course of the visit, I collected a great many other impressions and ideas that I have built upon in my subsequence palliative care activities and writings.

## INTRODUCING THE HOSPICE CONCEPT TO CROATIA

When I returned to Croatia, I wrote a letter that described my visit to St. Christopher's. This letter was published in a newspaper and drew the interest of some readers. Shortly thereafter, one of my former students in neurological electromyography discussed the possibilities of palliative care with me and then created the first hospital department for terminally ill patients. This unit was established in the rural town of Pozega.

A few months later, the Serbian/Yugoslav army started its aggression on Croatia. Desperate refugees flooded the nation by the hundreds of thousands. Hospitals and rehabilitation centers were overwhelmed by the number of wounded people. The mass media was filled with reports of killing, torture, revenge, and extreme suffering—physically, emotionally, socially, and spiritually.

The question was raised: does it make any sense to speak about "dying with dignity" amid so many terrible and extremely humiliating deaths? Is it realistic to speak about dying decently in a country where so many persons now cannot live decently?

The answer was positive. Yes, hospice philosophy and practice does make sense—as the counterpart, the response to the terror of the times, and as a spark that might activate the good features hidden in every human being!

The audience was shocked the first time I suggested that we discuss death. Very soon, however, I was invited to give lectures. Valuable support was offered by the Croatian Academy of Medical Sciences. The number of persons who wanted to be informed and involved in the project increased slowly, but steadily.

We used the following strategy. First, we surveyed the existence of related institutions and programs and the level of available information throughout Croatia. The results were very disappointing. The medical encyclopedia and its supplements, so thorough in most other respects, did not include the word "hospice." Medical students had never heard anything about how to approach the dying person. Nursing students had only a few hours of instruction on this topic.

The dominant opinion was that the suffering person should not be told the truth about the diagnosis and prognosis. It was clear that the dying person was very often isolated both physically and psychologically. At the same time, the newly established hospice unit had to close due to financial reasons and the insufficient education and support of the staff.

At this point, it seemed necessary to define the goals we had to reach. The first goal was to foster education regarding the nature of hospice/palliative care, and to do so both from the theoretical and the action or applied standpoint. Three types of activity were started: (1) organization of symposia; (2) establishment of The Croatian Society for Hospice/Palliative Care; (3) publication of articles and books; and (4) establishment of hospice units, including mobile teams.

## THE FIRST SYMPOSIA

The first symposium was held in Zagreb in May, 1994. Nigel Sykes of London was guest speaker for the introductory lecture. We then attempted to demonstrate the modern concept of hospice with a set of presentations by Croat specialists, who focused on their respective points of view on palliative care. Special attention was given to the issues of pain control and gastrointestinal symptomatology. The psychosocial aspects of palliative care were discussed in about a third of the presentations. The emphasis here was on communication, including ways of discussing diagnosis and prognosis and responding to bereavement and grief. Additionally, some sessions presented data about the relationship between terminal care practices and current societal attitudes toward death and dying.

The symposium organizers decided to continue with further hospice activities within the framework of the Croatian Hospice/Palliative Care Society. It may be of interest that four institutions cooperated in the organization of this symposium. The Croatian Academy of Medical Sciences was assisted by three citizen organizations: the Croatian League Against Cancer, and the Croatian-German and Croatian-American Associations.

A followup symposium was held in September, 1995, with quite a different profile. Presentations and round tables were devoted to selected topics such as children, HIV, Amyotropic Lateral Sclerosis (ALS) patients, spiritual aspects, pain control, communication, and pro- and contra-hospice. There were also teaching sessions with small group discussions and facilitators.

## THE CROATIAN SOCIETY FOR
## HOSPICE/PALLIATIVE CARE

During the first symposium, the decision was made to organize a society to promote the quality of life for terminally ill people with no regard to age, sex, race, religion, nationality, or personal resources. This goal is to be achieved through lectures, courses, symposia, and the publication of original or translated books on hospice/palliative care. A bulletin was also to provide informational articles on a regular basis. It was further decided that the Society should help to co-ordinate practitioners of the various specialties that are needed to deal with hospice/palliative care problems. Coordinative efforts should also be made to bring together the various institutions that are concerned with terminal care issues at home and abroad. Furthermore, the Society should differentiate between professional and personal criteria of the staff who provide services to terminally ill persons, and collaborate with existing physician organizations in supervising their activities and protecting both the care provider and the patient.

The regular members of the Society are physicians, specialists, and general practitioners. The associated members are nurses, psychologists, theologists, social workers, lawyers, pharmacists, physical therapists, and others who are qualified to help dying persons.

Founded in October, 1994, the Society now has about 70 members. Many guests also attend the monthly sessions and participate in round table discussions or other presentations. Two special working groups have started to address specific problems, such as providing care for children, and the selection and education of volunteers. This latter working group is active on the "grassroots" level.

## PUBLICATIONS

Three articles have already been published, and others are in press. Several books are also scheduled for publication in the near future, combining the contributions of palliative care specialists from Croatia and other parts of the world. For a complete list, please see Bibliography at the end of this chapter.

## FIRST ATTEMPTS TO ORGANIZE HOSPICE UNITS

Information and education are fundamental to the development of hospice/palliative care services in Croatia. This process should include sending interested younger collaborators to see how things are done abroad, but so far the shortage of funds has not made this approach possible.

We hope to organize the first home visiting team in the near future. This team will utilize volunteers who will work in connection with Mother Therese Sisters and the "Drop of Kindness" Catholic Society. We are also trying to establish the first rooms of a stationary unit that can provide services to terminally ill persons who lack financial resources and/or have no family care providers available.

Home visit services by general practitioners are subject to the extensive reorganization process that is occurring in Croatia's transition from a socialist to a market economy.

The entire process of establishing hospice/palliative care remains especially difficult while a state of war exists. We discuss ways of helping people end their lives in comfort and dignity, but the shells keep dropping.

God help us to endure!

## BIBLIOGRAPHY

### Published

Jusic, A. (1993). On death. *Acta Medica Croatica*, 47, 41–45.

Jusic, A. (1994). O hospicijima—Paliajativnoj skrbi u svijetu. *Lijecnicki Vjesnik*, 1–2, 46–47.

Poziac, V. (1993). Hospicij promice kulturu zivota. *Obnovljeni Zivot*, 5, 459–476.

### In Press

Jusic, A. Sto je to moderna hospicijska skrb ili palijativna medicina? *Lijecnicki Vjesnik*.

Jusic, A. Moderna hospicijska skrb ili palijativna medicina—Savremeni izazov. *Medicinski Glasni* (Osijek).

Jusic, A., & Sykes, N. The hospice movement in the world and its future in Croatia. *Acta Medica Croatica*.

# 12

# Hospice in France*

## Michele Salamagne

In the last century, a young French woman, Jeanne Gamier, lost her husband and her two children within a few months. This devastating experience led her to establish several hospitals for the care of the incurably ill. She was, indeed, carrying on a tradition dating back from the Middle Ages. These general hospitals were called "*Hotels-Dieu*" ("God's hostels.") A reminder of this tradition is the symbolic term "*hotels-Dieu*" ("God's houses") that has often been applied to general hospitals in France. The contemporary hospice movement in France, has arisen from this long tradition, but within the context of newly emerging social and medical conditions, as well as the continuing universal need to care for people in the last days of their lives.

## AT THE BEGINNING

### Influence of the British Hospice Movement

I started my career as an anesthesiologist in the 1970s. The techniques of intensive care had developed rapidly. Electronic monitoring of body functions, locoregional anesthesia, epidural catheters, and other new developments were changing our method of working.

* We appreciate the assistance of Benoit Ritzenthaler, M. D. (Myton Hamlet Hospice, Warwick, UK) in preparing the final draft of this chapter.

I became aware by hearsay of a British hospital where it was said that the patient's pain was eased through orally administered doses of diamorphine. This hospital was said to be the work of a woman doctor. Fact or rumor? A Jesuit father, P. Verspieren, director of a society of Catholic medical students in Paris, organized a study trip in 1975 and reported their observations on *"Therapeutiq des souffrances terminales"* (Therapy of terminal suffering) in a special issue of their publication. This information was circulated in French medical circles, but went almost unnoticed.

Pioneers who dared to ask pharmacists to prepare solutions of morphine chlorhydrate were met with resistance. (The use of diamorphine is prohibited by the French pharmacopoeia.) The pharmacists were reluctant to prepare what they regarded as a lethal elixir. They rejected prescriptions that would ease pain while enabling the terminally ill person to retain consciousness. Even when invited to read articles written by our British colleagues, the pharmacists remained unpersuaded.

At the time I was working in a small (100-bed) hospital in Paris. Here, the chief surgeon attached much importance to his patients' comfort. He considered that sick people should not only have surgical treatment, but should also be helped to remain comfortable with adequate analgesia if the cancer recurred. In such a favorable environment, I discovered that, when relieved from pain, patients can express themselves and air their feelings about their forthcoming death. The knowledge of morphine's metabolism and its ability to relieve pain effectively made me feel really good and efficient. However, I was not prepared for the new opening into existential illness and spiritual distress that pain relief allowed.

## A Canadian Connection

Meanwhile, on the other side of the ocean, our French-speaking Canadian friends in Montreal were organizing a congress on palliative care, supervised by Dr. Balfour Mount, who had previously benefitted from contacts with Dr. Cicely Saunders and St. Christopher's Hospice. From 1978 onwards, I attended the Montreal Congress for Palliative Care, held every other year. These meetings gave me the opportunity to learn from the experience of our Canadian friends, gather specialized journals, and meet colleagues who told me about their palliative care units. I was dreaming of establishing such a unit in my own hospital and came back in 1980 with a useful book, *The R. V. H. Manual on Palliative Hospice Care.*

In February, 1978, the Laennec Center invited Professor. Mount to Paris. He spoke to an audience of anaesthetsts and intensive care doctors about the concept of palliative care. They were much more interested in central neurological path-ways than in the absorption of a simple mixture. This first meeting was rather controversial, but the academic background of Professor. Mount (McGill University) gave a significant weight to the new ideas.

## Therese Vanier

Another doctor decided to enter the crusade. Dr. Therese Vanier had worked at St. Christopher's Hospice and spoke French perfectly. She contributed to our efforts from October, 1976 onward. She was invited to speak at a large hospital in Paris, but had difficulty in convincing her audience. Despite the disheartening beginning, numerous invitations were to follow in the subsequent decade. Dr. Vanier proved to be a straightforward and determined orator who vividly conveyed how a patient could take advantage of simple and efficient methods of treatment.

She was the voice of St. Christopher's Hospice team, and brought us their support and encouragement. She familiarized us with the latest research carried out by Dr. Saunders' team, and stimulated us to undertake our own studies. Dr. Vanier also suggested that I translate Saunders' and Baines' book, *Living and Dying*. The French edition that came out in 1986 borrowed its title from the poet Jacques Prevert: "*La vie est dans la Mort*" (Life is in death). A second edition was to follow up dating to the basic information. In 1988, I contributed to the French version of C. Regnard and A. Davies' guideline book, *Symptom Relief in Advanced Cancer*. This book, republished in 1994, is much appreciated by French general practitioners.

## The First French Associations of Palliative Care

University circles remained impervious to the concept of palliative care. However, committed supporters were to be found beyond the enclosures of hospitals. Many ordinary citizens also joined representatives of the medical profession to form several associations.

JALMALV (initials of the French words, *Jusqu' a La Mort Accompagner la Vie*: "Watching over life until the moment of death") was founded in 1983. It soon became a national federation of more than 50 associations and more than 4,000 members throughout the whole country. Other associations spruing up in Paris with similar or complementary purposes. These included ASP (*Association pour les Soins Palliatifs*—Association for Palliative Care), *Fonction Soignante et Accompagnement* (Nursing and Supporting Patients), and *Vieillir Ensemble* (Growing Old Together).

Further afield throughout France, many more associations have flourished. Our country is presently covered with a dense network of associations that support the development of palliative care. Most of these associations are aligned with "La Société Française de Soins Palliatifs (French Society for Palliative Care)," whose main function is to represent them to the French government and to European authorities.

# THE TURNING POINT

In 1984 a proeuthanasia wave swept through France. An opinion poll published in a daily medical newspaper stated that 24% of general practitioners supported active euthanasia by lethal injections. The routine use of lytic cocktails in hospitals also came to light, thanks to the publication of an article by Patrick Verspieren in the January 1984 issue of the journal, *Etudes*. These concoctions are, unfortunately, still used in some units nowadays. They are made up of a mixture of chlorpromazine (Thorazine), pethidine, and prometazine in an IV solution. A film demonstrating the practice of euthanasia was shown to a very enthusiastic audience at a conference of "Association Pour le Droit de Mourir dans la Dignité" (Association for the Right to Die in Dignity). Very few dared to condemn this act. The news hit the headlines, and euthanasia seemed to be the only solution when "there was nothing else to do."

The National Advisory Ethics Committee was created in the same year. A number of voices arose in the media to express a different point of view. They maintained that the dilemma is not achoice between artificial prolongation of life by medical means and euthanasia, but that palliative care represented a valid third alternative.

As a result of public concern, the State Secretary of Health called an interdisciplinary working group to look at the circumstances surrounding the end of life. The report of this group was published in 1985: *Soigner et Accompagner Jusqu'au Bour* (Patient Care and Support to the Very End). This most significant document meant the official commission of palliative care in France. The following extract gives a flavor of its importance: "It is essential that the health authorities ensure that, at the end of life, each individual has a right to respect, dignity, relief of suffering and medical care adapted to every stage, especially at the time of death."

## The Consequences

From then on, everything went very fast. The first palliative care unit opened in 1987 at Paris University City Hospital under the direction of Dr. Abiven.

The trustees in charge of the Paris state-owned hospital system, that constitutes the largest medical establishment in Europe (50 hospitals, 750 ward units and 85,000 employees), envisaged a combined plan of action. On the one hand, they were to set up outpatient departments where people could receive medical care and information about palliative care, and, on the other hand, they were to establish inpatient pallaitive care units.

The first premises were opened at the Hotel-Dieu Hospital. The second unit opened at Paul Brousee Hospital where Dr. Renée Sebag had been working for several years for the care and dignity of dependent and very old patients. I was given the opportunity to work by her side and take the medical responsibility for the palliative care unit that she was to open and manage.

## FAREWELL TO ANESTHESIA: FULL TIME PALLIATIVE CARE BEGINS

At that time, a new team was to take over from the retiring senior surgeon in the hospital where I had been working for 18 years. Beside running the anesthesia and intensive care departments, I had set up a palliative care outpatient consultation. I dreamt of creating a palliative care unit in this hospital, but the new managerial team was not convinced, despite the satisfaction expressed by patients and families, the support of Dr. Vanier, and the enthusiasm of the nonmedical staff. Unfortunately, back in 1989, the establishment was not ready to welcome such a program. I had to accept defeat, despite my militancy, and therefore decided to leave.

I was delighted to meet new challenges away from the operating room and intensive care cubicles. I was looking for the words patients had lost because of their physical pain and global suffering. The long wait since I had first become interested in palliative care in 1977 suddenly began to make sense. During that time, I had been given many opportunities—becoming familiar with new treatments, getting involved in associations promoting palliative care, taking part in numerous teaching sessions for nurses, volunteers, and occasionally doctors, and learning to write articles for professional and lay medical journals. During that time, I also came to appreciate the pitfalls of media interviews, and learned to analyze my own attraction to this world of the extreme.

I knew that I had to leave the comforting and concrete world of surgery and intensive care that was so full of speed and action. Taking part in this new adventure was also a family choice. I involved my husband and children, who were living in tune with my joys, struggles, and bereavements. Despite a shade of fear or sometimes disapproval from our friends, my own family gave me unconditional support.

## Starting the Palliative Care Project

The first step was to appoint a multidisciplinary caring team. The hospital management board agreed to the following organization chart:

- A full-time doctor in charge of the team, with 4 part-time medical practitioners;
- A medical house officer with full-time secretarial support;

- Fourteen registered nurses, eight nurse auxiliaries, and two technicians, led by a nurse in charge;
- A part-time psychologist and a part-time social worker;
- A physiotherapist and a dietician; and
- A Catholic chaplain and a number of volunteers.

Architects were contacted to convert one of the buildings within the 800-bed Paul Brousse Hospital. After only a few meetings with the multidisciplinary team, a group of architects was selected from those who had been newly certified. Their plans showed their inventive spirit. They took advantage of the structure to leave bare stone within the building, while large windows produced a bright and warm atmosphere. Every space available was adapted into meeting areas for caregivers, families, and visitors. The passages became encounter areas, where the caregivers, families and visitors could see each other. Particular attention was given to the design of consulting rooms that give the feeling of a homelike atmosphere, in contrast with the traditional hospital setting.

Families had their own premises which included a kitchen, dining room, living room, and bedrooms. The welcoming atmosphere was enhanced by a pleasant garden just outside each patient's bedroom.

Unfortunately, with time, we discovered many pitfalls in this lovely and innovative design, such as inappropriate use of materials for roofing, the outside walls, and the floors. The young designers' lack of experience led to the problem that windows and doors were not adapted to wheelchairs. Furthermore, the attractive layout did not take into account quality insulation and soundproof walls. With the advantage of hindsight, I advise those who have the opportunity to contribute to the building of a new unit to visit other units to help foresee possible difficulties. We found that the building should facilitate the work of the multidisciplinary team, besides guaranteeing quality care. The palliative care philosophy should rule the architecture of the unit.

## Nurse Manager and Doctor in Charge

The consultant in charge of our department had the responsibility of choosing both the nurse manager and doctor in charge. We did not know each other, and it took some time to begin to work as a team. We had to take into account our weaknesses and strengths and respect each other's area of responsibility. We found that a partnership had to be worked out meticulously. Our team, like others, went through crises, but the leaders were able to see each other through, since they did not feel seriously wounded. We negotiated essential issues, such as the respective place of doctors and nurses in the organization, the role of the psychologist, the details of job descriptions, the working hours, and even the choice of furniture and equipment. This negotiation process made our projects clearer and pulled us together.

## Initial Team Training

We were fortunate enough to be able to set aside a full month for the initial training of the team. All team members had their say regarding organization, philosophy of care, complementary therapies, and ongoing training. During this first month, we had the opportunity to share our views on many issues such as flextime, welcoming of patients and families, differential roles of trained nurses and auxiliaries, personal views on euthanasia, and much more. Time went very fast, and this period remains a stimulating memory for all those who participated. Since then, every new member of the team is allowed a full month for the initial training prior to being operational.

## Computerization of Patients' Files

From the very beginning, we decided to enter all our care plans and medical assessments on computer. Since February 12, 1990, the memory of our unit has been growing on the computer's hard disk (nicknamed "chouchou," or, in English, "darling.") Only minimum daily observations are committed to paper. There is easy access to the computer, so that everyone in the team can acquire a comprehensive knowledge of the patient, including nursing, medical, and psychological aspects.

Keyboarding, however, is not the only means of communication. There is a staff meeting twice a day to go over patient care. After all these years, we have collected a very large amount of data that would be available for clinical research. It is a pity that current budget restrictions do not allow us to make use of the data accumulated over that time. With hindsight, we now see that research should have been part of the unit philosophy from the beginning.

## Volunteers

Our intention from the beginning was to ask volunteers to cooperate with the work of professionals. However, the latter were not prepared for this partnership at that time. Professionals feared the possibility of losing their predominant roles at the patient's bedside, and saw volunteers as invaders. This reluctance was hidden behind obscure explanations, for example, "wanting to find their feet" before introducing volunteer staff.

After a delay of 6 months, the team finally accepted the introduction of a few volunteers. These were four experienced people who had worked for some years in geriatrics and kept themselves extremely discrett. Everyone was—mutually—

on their guard, but the number of volunteers slowly increased, each person bringing specific skills, such as craft work, to the task.

After three years, the volunteers took a higher profile, leading their own association, which has a contractual agreement with the hospital management. The criteria for acceptance are stringent. For instance, volunteers have to have two interviews with psychologists prior to being accepted for training. They find out about their future tasks in a gradual, sequential manner, and are integrated into a group run by a volunteer coordinator. The volunteers-in-training are accompanied by an experienced volunteer when they are first introduced to patients and families. After a while, they are allowed to be on duty alone. At the moment we have 30 volunteers who share their work in shifts of four to five hours each day, from 9 a.m. to 10 p.m.

Volunteers attend regular training sessions on subjects such as music therapy, how to listen to patients, and touch and communication skills. They also attend university hospital lectures with great enthusiasm. Regular meetings are held with a psychologist who has no other link with the hospital, and they also have the opportunity to share their experiences with fellow volunteers in the absence of any members of the professional team. The volunteers have now been well accepted by the professional members of the multidisciplinary team, who recognize their beneficial contributions to patients and families.

## Spiritual Care

We recognize that patients and families have a religious need. The contribution of our chaplain, Eliane, is very valuable. She is fully in tune with the staff and attends our afternoon meetings prior to visiting patients. However, clergy are not automatically welcome in a state hospital, given that the democratic constitution of France clearly separates the State and the Church. Moreover, the religious beliefs of our team members themselves range across a wide spectrum from atheism to deep commitment, while the majority have no particular religious affiliation.

## Clinical Activity and Patient Profile

Over a period of slightly less than five years, 531 patients received care in the unit, 62 of whom were admitted on more than one occasion. Some were transferred to other wards to benefit from specific therapies. Most patients suffered from cancer (85%). AIDS (14%) and degenerative neurological disease (1%) were the conditions afflicting other patients. The mean age of cancer patients was 61, and only 35 for AIDS patients. The average length of stay was 22 days for cancer patients and 31 for AIDS patients.

We find that the care of patients suffering from cancer and AIDS is quite different, not only because of the specific knowledge required in oncology and infectious disease, but also because of the wide disparity in social background.

Most patients suffering with a terminal illness are cared for in ordinary hospital wards. We are called on for advice on very difficult cases when hospital teams are struggling. Patients who request euthanasia often are referred to us. Our intervention must be very effective to change attitudes and raise new hopes. Some patients have nowhere to go, being foreigners without work permits, or political refugees awaiting recognition.

Some patients have become impoverished as a result of their illness, and sometimes though the rejection of families who refuse to acknowledge and speak the name of their "long-lasting and disabling illness," i. e., AIDS.

Confrontated with such extreme poverty, we tend to call our government health care policy into question. Deprivation occurs particularly with those who do not speak our language and/or have beliefs that are totally unknown to us. Howe can we break their isolation and respond to their need? The precariousness of human life is so vividly present in a person's last days. How can we understand another's suffering while we ourselves have to face our own distress in those circumstances? The close relationship with the dying person makes us feel more vulnerable and, therefore, possibly more human. We need time to recover and refill ourselves with joy.

## Bereavement Service

Bereaved relatives and friends are invited by our psychologist to attend small discussion groups twice monthly. Most participants had a relative who died on the unit. They are given the opportunity of describing their coping efforts, expressing their grief, and planning their lives beyond the difficult period they are experiencing. Some of the relatives who have been through this healing process return to contribute further to these meetings.

## Preadmission Consultation

Preadmission consultation was established at the beginning of the unit and remains an essential component of care. Away from hospital activity, time seems to stop for a while, so that patients, families, and staff can get to know each other. Patients have the opportunity to share their understanding of the disease and express their needs.

It is a moment when they can think about how they want to organize the rest of their lives and what they want to share with relatives and close friends. We want to know what they authorize us to tell families and friends and to whom it is more appropriate to do so. Sometimes the preadmission consulting situation provides a forum for patients and relatives to express their fear, anger, regrets, and guilt or, more positively, their hopes, dreams, and fantasies. Through attentive listening we get to know the patient, and this is likely to improve our ability to provide a high quality of care while the patient is in the unit.

The consultation is carried out jointly by the nurse and the doctor who serve as team representatives. We explain our method of working, the role of each staff member, our aims, and ethics. Sometimes patients expect to be "helped on the way to death." Our reply is that we do not practice euthanasia, but are truly open to hear their requests on days of despair. In such circumstances we find that the approaches of the nurses and doctors are very much complementary. Patients and families are then given the opportunity to have a look at the unit and see the room that will be allocated to the patient (this is not an obligation, but an invitation).

The preadmission consultation takes two to three hours. The average specialist consultation, by contrast, lasts about 15 minutes. The time required to allow patients to express their needs is difficult to convey in the coldness of statistical terms and figures. We have to explain our methods and aims to each new administrator. We do not want to be mistaken for or compared with a curative unit, since the palliative care service is of another kind.

## Communication Within the Team

The day and the night teams exchange information every morning and every evening. Of course, our darling *couchou* is watching, and is always ready to tell the story of a patient when required. Nurses and auxiliaries pass on what the patients have said. It is essential to recognize the difference between a private conversation, what can be entered on the computer, and what should be passed on by word of mouth. We need to strike the right balance between effective communication and respect for the patient's privacy.

During the report, doctors are asked to explain their prescribed treatment and the reason for drug changes. Sometimes changes are suggested by the team. We all need to develop a good listening ear and the capacity to define the real needs of patients. Doctors are encouraged to listen to suggestions with an open mind and, in case of difficulties, to discuss them with medical colleagues working in the unit. The role of each member of the palliative care team has been brought up many times in our discussion group, and questions have apparently been resolved with the agreement of all. However, in practice, this question remains a constant source of difficulties. The multidisciplinary approach is a school of mutual respect and a requirement of true palliative care provision.

In addition to team meetings, doctors have a session once a week to review patient care, critically evaluate the treatment, and plan for the next few days. A summary of the meeting is added to the computer record in each patient's file and is available to all members of the team. Originally, there was no purely medical meeting, but we found these necessary to improve medical care and define the specific role of doctors within the multidisciplinary team.

## The Discussion Group

This group is open to all permanent paid staff and is led by a psychoanalyst, who offered this service since the opening of the unit. He has no knowledge of the patients except through what is said in the group. Out of 35 team members, 10 devotees attend every Wednesday meeting. Where are the others? Probably, some do not like the psychoanalyst's approach and other have been "draft-dodgers" since the beginning.

The group members discuss what they perceive as specific difficulties over broad areas of interest in order to improve their knowledge of the patients and families. The content of these meetings is strictly confidential. Of course, it is not our intention to analyze the personality of our patients, but rather to bring to light information that could be of benefit to the whole unit, both patients and caregivers. Night staff also have their discussion group once a month, with the same psychoanalyst, during working hours.

## The Terminal Care Support Team

From the beginning, we have visited hospital patients at the invitation of the medical team in charge. Progressively, the initial opposition toward palliative care has disappeared. Oncology and internal medicine staff who attended the university degree course have acted as facilitators of an improved approach to the relief of suffering. At the infectious disease unit, they often ask us to step in when patients are in extreme pain. These calls are often prompted as much by the team's suffering as the patient's pain. We try to decipher the motivation that originates these crises. It is not possible to unfreeze a difficult situation by a quick phone call on how to adjust a morphine dose.

There is a real danger of falling into the grap of excessive activity to the detriment of the essentials of palliative care—listening, nonjudgmental approach, respect, and ethical thinking. For two years, one of our doctors had been attending the oncology staff meeting. After reflection, we decided to withdraw this commitment, since we realized it was worsening the opposition to our palliative care program. Our way of dealing with patients' pain without causing loss of consciousness has been perceived as "officious active treatment in incurable cases," which many have accused oncologists of practising. Since our views on terminal care are so different from those of our oncologist colleagues, we have decided to respond to referrals from them by offering palliative care consultations within our unit. By withdrawing into our territory, we feel that we can protect each other's identity.

## The Teaching Commitment

Teaching is an essential part of our activity. Most of our trainees are nurses. They come to work alongside us for one week at a time. These are mainly nurses, who have been working for years as managers or tutors. Occasionally we also have psychologists, physiotherapists, and volunteers. Sometimes doctors who are studying for their university diploma spend a week with us to gain some practical experience. As a matter of policy we allow ourselves one week a month without any trainees to give us the opportunity to spend some time among ourselves. This monthly "holiday time" considerably lightens our load. It is hard to keep this time free, because training is more and more requested. We now have to plan training arrangements at least 6 months in advance.

Since 1990 we have offered a university course that provides lectures one evening a week on various subjects related to palliative care. The students are doctors, postgraduate medical students, nurses, psychologists, and volunteers who already have some involvement in palliative care.

During last year's course, we allocated time for discussion. The students spoke of the difference between what is taught to them and what is the current clinical practice in their own units. The gap is sometimes too wide for them. They report finding themselves in unmanageable situations, and therefore welcome the opportunity to talk about it with fellow students. Because this sharing process proved to be so useful, the discussion meetings were repeated this year.

Doctors, nurses, auxiliary nurses, and psychologists of the unit are often asked to give courses or lecture in universities, nursing colleges, schools of social work, and to volunteer groups. They are also asked to take part in public debates or to give testimony on the radio or television. We were first very enthusiastic about these contacts with the media. As we became more experienced, however, we learned to be cautious and avoid being involved in an emotional approach that might have negative connotations for some people. The complexity of the feelings of a person in great difficulty does not lend itself to the bustle and pressure of a recording studio. Fortunately, though, some journalists have turned away from sensationalism, and have contributed much to a better public perception of the role of palliative care by producing highly sensitive television programs.

## IF WE HAD TO DO IT AGAIN?

Without any hesitation, I would leave again for a new crusade to live this adventure, to know the beginnings of the associative circles which built a sound foundation for an official policy making on palliative care. The structures development in our country was amazing: from no units in 1986 to 26 in 1992 (356 beds) and 37 in 1995 (430 beds). There were no terminal care support teams in

1986, 6 in 1992, and 35 in 1996. I was present at the inception of *Palliative Care University* degree. There are 15 nowadays in the whole territory, starting from nothing in 1989.

From this year, teaching of palliative care is compulsory for medical students, and their practice is considered as essential by our new professional code of ethics.

Living and working in our palliative care unit has been a great experience for me. I have been delighted to work towards building up a team and developing a good atmosphere. I have learned a great deal in the clinical field and in dealing with crises. I have developed many commitments in associations and in the teaching world.

Although I maintain that life should be preserved, I have not been so kind with my own. I have let my professional life overflow into my personal time. I need to make new choices and regain some freedom outside palliative care.

So, if I had to do it again, I would encourage myself to say "no" without feeling guilty, since I am firmly convinced that my psychological and physical health is priceless. That would mean cutting my commitments by half. However, since I cannot turn the clock back, I would like to advise those who seek to launch such a project: "Take time. It is by taking time that you will be in tune with what is the true essence of palliative care."

# REFERENCES

Ajemian, I., & Mount, B. (Eds.) (1980). *The RVH manual on palliative hospice care.* New York: Arno Press.

Delbecque, R. (1994). *Les soins palliatifs et l'accompagnement des malades en fin de vie.* Paris: La Documentation Française.

Regnard, C. F. B., & Davies, A. (1986). *A guide to symptom relief in advanced cancer.* Manchester, England: Haigh and Hochland.

Salamagne, M. H. (1993). Le traitement de la douleur cancereuse chronique. *La Revue du Praticien: Médecine Generale, 7,* 15–21.

Salamagne, M. H., & Hirsch, E. (1992). *Accompagner jusqu'au bout de la vie.* Paris: Cerf.

Salamagne, M. H., & Vanier, T. (1986). Douleur physique, souffrance globale a la phase ultime d'une maladie cancereuse. *La Revue du Praticien, 36,* 457–469.

Saunders, C. (1978). *The management of terminal disease.* London: Edward Arnold.

Saunders, C., & Baines, M. (1983). *Living with dying.* Oxford: Oxford University Press.

Sebag-Lanoe, R. (1986). *Mourir accompagne.* Paris: Desclee de Brouwer.

Vespiren, P. (1984). *Face a celui qui meurt.* Paris: Desclee de Brouwer.

# 13

# Hospice in Great Britain

## Avril Jackson and Ann Eve

This chapter is written from the perspective of the Hospice Information Service, an international link and resource for members of the public and health professionals, and part of St. Christopher's Hospice since 1977. During this time, we have witnessed a great change in attitude and practice toward care of the dying patients and their families, in step with the remarkable development of the hospice movement both in the United Kingdom and Ireland and throughout the world. For several years the Information Service was the only source of information for those wishing to find out more about hospice care or, indeed, how to start a hospice.

Hospice and palliative care is not the exclusive province of any single provider. A range of agencies offer different types of care for different needs. In addition, the modern hospice movement is underpinned by a growing body of research, several journals, and, currently, 16 professional associations which facilitate communication and support the work of doctors, nurses, social workers, and other disciplines. Hospices and palliative care services in Britain now care for well over half of all patients dying of cancer, and the basic philosophy of palliative care is being applied more widely to include people with other terminal illnesses, such as motor neuron disease and AIDS.

The word *hospice* was first used from the 4th century onwards, when Christian orders welcomed travelers, the sick, and those in need. It was first applied to the care of dying patients by Madame Jeanne Garnier, who founded the Dames de Calvaire in Lyon, France, in 1842. Other religious institutions, such as The Irish

Sisters of Charity at Our Lady's Hospice in Dublin (1879) also cared for the dying. The idea was further developed by the same order at St. Joseph's Hospice in London (1905), where later Dame Cicely Saunders was to carry out her early research into the control of pain. In the 1950s, the Marie Curie Memorial Foundation (now Marie Curie Cancer Care) established eleven nursing homes throughout the country to care for patients with terminal cancer in response to a nationwide survey which revealed poor quality of care for patients with cancer who were being nursed at home. But it was the founding of St. Christopher's Hospice in Southeast London in 1967 that spearheaded the development of the modern Hospice movement. St. Christopher's was the first hospice to bring the academic model of research and teaching together with clinical care for people with far advanced disease.

## HOSPICE INPATIENT CARE

The first decade of the modern hospice movement saw a steady increase in the number of hospices, but this growth was almost exclusively confined to inpatient hospice services. Economically, it was a period of relative affluence. The trend was for buildings, and most services were initiated by local communities that identi- fied the need for a hospice and raised the necessary funds for the capital costs and for ongoing operations. These voluntary and independent hospices were regis- tered charities, receiving varying amounts from their local National Health Service regional health authorities. Their economic survival was often dependent almost completely on local goodwill and fundraising initiatives.

Not until 1988 was there any centrally provided funding for which all hospices were eligible, although in practice this support was unevenly distributed. The overall amount has been increased annually, and currently the voluntary hospices receive about 60 million pounds, which is about 25% of their total running costs. In addition, a program has been introduced whereby hospices are able to receive free supplies of drugs, to the value of about 6 million pounds.

Increased government support and recognition are due largely to the efforts of the charity "Help the Hospice," and to the subsequent creation in 1991 of the National Council for Hospice and Specialist Palliative Care Services, which con- tinues to be the representative body for all hospice and palliative care services in England, Wales, and Northern Ireland. The National Hospice Council has set up several working parties to examine crucial aspects of hospice and palliative care: euthanasia, quality of care, research, pain in advanced cancer, education, access to palliative care services by members of black and ethnic minority communities, standards and definitions, and collection of minimum data. A range of useful publications is now available. The Hospice Information Service has a good working relationship with the National Hospice Council and is currently collaborating in a joint data collection project. Similar organizations to the National Hospice Council exist in Scotland and the Republic of Ireland.

Despite greater government recognition, however, funding remains precarious. Consequently, voluntary hospices continue to rely enormously on public goodwill and the ingenuity and steadfastness of local supporters who jump from high buildings, utilize miles of knitting yarn, shave their heads, and engage in countless other sponsored fundraising activities in the name of hospice! Indeed, donations and legacies are vital to the survival of the hospice community, accounting for 66% of total income. A further source of income for many voluntary hospices is the charity shop, which sells donated secondhand and nearly new goods, ranging from books, bric-a-brac, household items, and even castoff designer clothes! One hospice charity shop in the Northeast, situated in a prime position near the port, counts among its regular customers visiting seamen from eastern Europe and Africa. But financial gain is only part of the benefit. The fundraising effort can also provide a focus for the hospice in its local community and increase public awareness, not only of the individual hospice, but of the whole kaleidoscope of hospice care. Although most shops are managed by a salaried staff member, the workforce is provided by volunteers who often have an association with the hospice, frequently through personal bereavement. For them, the companionship and support of other volunteers in the hospice shop can be very important, and equally valued is their understanding welcome to people who come in to the shop with items no longer required by a lost relative.

In 1975 the first of the National Health Service continuing care units opened, initiated by the Relief Macmillan fund, the national cancer charity. This development set the pattern for some dozen hospices, whereby the charity provided capital funding for units built in the grounds of NHS hospitals, with agreement that the NHS would subsequently provide the running costs. By the late 1970s, there were about 60 hospice inpatient units. At the present time (1996) there are just over 200 hospice and palliative care inpatient services in the UK, providing over 3,000 beds. The growth in the last 15 years has been in the number of services (a 3.5-fold increase), rather than in the number of beds, which have increased by a factor of less than 2.5. This implies that the trend has been towards smaller hospices. In fact, the most common size for a hospice is 10 beds, while the average number of beds is 15. About 18% of the 160,000 people dying of cancer each year in the UK do so in a hospice or palliative care unit. Rather more than this number, however, actually receive some care within a unit, as nearly half of all admissions result in discharge after symptom control, but only 25% of admissions are readmissions. The implications are that many of those discharged actually die at home or elsewhere outside of hospice facilities.

## HOME CARE SERVICES

Many patients with terminal illness wish to remain at home for as long as possible, and nearly two-thirds of the cancer patients who die each year receive some care from hospice or palliative home care services that work alongside GPs and the primary healthcare team. Nurses work in an advisory and supportive capacity, providing information on pain and symptom control as well as giving emotional support both to patients and carers.

The first home care team was pioneered by St. Christopher's Hospice in 1969. Six years later, the first Macmillan Service was established at St. Joseph's Hospice in east London, but it was not until the late 1970s that the first of the community Macmillan Nurses were appointed. There are now over 1,000 Macmillan Nurses working in hospitals, hospices, and in the community as part of the NHS. There are currently 384 home care teams in the UK and Ireland. There are also some 5,000 Marie Curie Nurses, who care for patients at home day and night. This service is run in conjunction with the district nursing service in most health authorities. Respite Care at Home, or Hospice at Home, is a further more recent initiative that enables patients to stay at home longer and lighten the load on caregivers and often avoid admission to an inpatient unit. There are currently about 50 such services attached to British hospices where a multiprofessional team, with access to consultant advice, offers a comprehensive 24-hour service, including practical nursing and night sitting. The team may also be supported by experienced volunteers.

## HOSPICE IN A HOSPITAL SETTING

Another area in which there has been significant development in the past 10–15 years is the provision of hospital-based services. The concept of the hospital support team, pioneered in the UK in 1976 by St. Thomas's Hospital, London, was similar to the team which originated at St. Luke's Hospital, New York in 1974. This was a multiprofessional team of doctors, nurses, social worker, chaplain, and secretary, a configuration that frequently has been emulated elsewhere to provide symptom control, pain relief, and emotional support to patients and caregivers. The trend now appears to be for the appointment of a single nurse who may not only visit patients on the wards, but also work more within the oncology departments, seeing patients from point of diagnosis right through the course of their illness. In some cases, contact is continued when a patient is discharged into the community. About 250 hospitals in the United Kingdom now have such support services.

Calls to the Information Service poignantly remind us of the importance of such services for large hospitals for people who have been recently diagnosed with cancer and are alone and bewildered. Simply providing the name of the right person or team can often be the vital key to unlocking further resources and receiving clear, understandable explanations.

## HOSPICE DAY CARE

Perhaps the most dramatic increase has been in the availability of day care. This type of service was almost nonexistent 15 years ago but now is provided by more than 220 programs. About two-thirds are attached to hospice inpatient units and the remainder are freestanding. Day care is an important supplement to home care services that allows patients to continue living at home while maintaining contact with all the hospice facilities.

A wide range of creative and social activities is provided. Some services include medical and nursing care, physiotherapy, occupational therapy, hairdressing, chiropody, and beauty treatments. For many patients the creative activities—painting, writing, drawing, cooking, working with clay—offered by the day center provide an opportunity to regain some element of control and confidence, as well as to develop new ways of thinking about their situation. An exhibition of paintings, pottery, quilting, and weaving by patients attending the Day Centre at St. Christopher's Hospice was recently held in London. The medical director of the Marie Curie Centre in Liverpool remarked, "It is a demonstration of the creativity of people at a stage in their lives which is more commonly associated with dependency and lack of achievement."

## VOLUNTEERS

It is often said that the hospice movement, with its sometimes precarious level of funding, owes its existence to volunteers. An estimated (and this is possibly a conservative estimate) 30,000 volunteers work in British hospices. There can be very few jobs within the hospice context which are not being done somewhere by a volunteer. Like the other professional associations, the Association of Hospice Voluntary Service Coordinators is concerned to identify and maintain good practice in the management of volunteers and to ensure their successful integration into the workforce. Recruitment, selection, and support of volunteers is clearly of paramount importance, and it is encouraging that one British hospice has recently won a prestigious award for its training excellence. This clearly innovative hospice is also due to make its first volunteer exchange in the autumn with volunteers from a French palliative care service.

# EDUCATION AND TRAINING

Palliative care is now taught to many doctors and nurses in their training, and palliative medicine is increasingly integrated with mainstream medicine. In 1987, palliative medicine was recognized by the Royal College of Physicians as a specialty within general medicine, and there are currently four professors of palliative medicine in Great Britain. Most of the larger hospices provide an education service and offer conferences and seminars on palliative care and bereavement. Inquiries about educational opportunities frequently come to the Hospice Information Service, and since 1986 we have published a nationwide listing of courses, conferences, and seminars. Such is the demand and diversity that we now publish an update every six weeks and include major events overseas.

Many years ago the founder of the modern hospice movement, Dame Cicely Saunders, said that hospices needed to develop outside the NHS "so that attitudes and knowledge could move back in." There is now much evidence that the philosophy and principles of palliative care have impinged on many different settings and have done much to improve standards of care for dying patients and their families throughout the world. You have only to spend a little time in the Hospice Information Service to appreciate this contribution at firsthand, for the calls come in thick and fast: The primary school teacher overwhelmed by the imminent death of a five-year-old's mother: how will she support the little girl—and are there any books suitable for the 29 classmates? The policeman responsible for training: how can he prepare his staff to break bad news? The nurse from New York whose patient just wants to go home to die: is there a hospice in Nigeria? The concerned staff nurse from a busy oncology ward in an NHS hospital; can you suggest any helpful resources for my patients and relatives?

In one way or another, each of these issues is addressed by those engaged in hospice and palliative care, thanks to a remarkable sharing of knowledge and experience. Perhaps one of the simplest but most positive things about our work in the Hospice Information Service is being able to say "Yes, there is someone who can help."

Education and training in palliative care was always part of the vision of St. Christopher's. A formal program of education began in 1973, with the opening of the Study Centre. As the first teaching and research hospice, it soon began to attract other pioneering hospice workers who looked to St. Christopher's for guidance and, with growing professional and public awareness, for general information on the nature and provision of other hospice services around the country. In 1977, our work in responding to the many inquiries was formalized in the shape of a national Hospice Information Service.

Although St. Christopher's has been ever willing to share its knowledge and experience, it was never the intention to create a prescriptive, "Big Brother" type of organization. What we perceived to be important—and still do—was the networking: the building of links with others engaged in what was then a fairly fringe area of medicine and social care. Our mandate was also to collect and disseminate the experiences of others, so that people in the early stages of planning a hospice might avoid "reinventing the wheel." Our series of *Fact Sheets* on various aspects of hospice planning and management and useful facts and figures are attempts to respond to the questions we so frequently receive: "How do you start a hospice home care team?", "What equipment do you need in a physiotherapy department?", or "How many patients are cared for by palliative care services?" There is no single blueprint to starting a hospice, but the *Fact Sheets* can sometimes be a useful starting point for further discussion.

As hospice development filtered across the world it became apparent that we had an international, as well as a national role, to play. The Study Centre of St. Christopher's has had much contact with people who came for clinical experience or training and who subsequently return to their own countries to adapt principles and skills of hospice care to suit local needs. For many care providers, a membership with the Hospice Information Service provides a continuing link, a means of keeping up to date with developments in palliative care, and a sense of communality not readily available in their own locales. This is especially true for people from developing countries where resources are so often scarce and a sense of isolation difficult to avoid. A membership with the Hospice Information Service provides a continuing link, and a means of keeping up to date with developments in palliative care.

Our newsletter, the *Hospice Bulletin*, reflects hospice and palliative care activity throughout the world and for many of the newer services it can provide a sort of "shop window" in which to promote their development and achievements and sometimes to share problems. As well as many reports from the more established initiatives recent issues have included glimpses of the difficulties (and considerable achievements!) in setting up services in less well-resourced countries including Croatia, Romania, Russia, Africa, and India. A further useful resource to health care workers planning visits to the United Kingdom is our publication, *Choices*, listing upcoming courses and conferences on palliative care and bereavement.

St. Christopher's continues to make a significant contribution to the world of Hospice Care, particularly through its education program which includes an excellent library with access to over 5,000 books and articles on palliative care and bereavement and a specialist course for doctors from countries with a developing palliative are service as well as by the many lectures overseas undertaken by our staff. However, we are by no means unique in our commitment to hospice care in other countries. There is growing awareness and interest among hospice personnel in the UK in overseas hospice and palliative care development, as well as a willingness to share. A recent survey by the Hospice Information Service into Hospice Twinning revealed an encouraging amount of interaction between the UK: 13 "Hospice Twins," 10 academic links, and around 30 informal links between British and overseas hospices. A variety of support was offered, including local fundraising initiatives, exporting unused drugs, a shared research newsletter, staff and volunteer exchanges, correspondence exchange, purchase of equipment and supplies, training, and clinical placements. The survey also identified a total of 24 different languages spoken by British hospice staff and volunteers, which has enabled us to help overseas services locate an appropriate contributor for training purposes.

Several organizations have been set up specifically to address the needs of hospices in developing countries. The International School for Cancer Care, a British-based charity under the leadership of Dr. Robert Twycross, has for several years provided advice and training for people from overseas for whom education and training in palliative cancer care is not readily available in their own countries. The Sheffield-based British Aid for Hospices Abroad (BAHA) includes a multiprofessional group of hospice personnel with an interest in identifying ways of contributing towards the development of hospice care in Eastern Europe.

Other groups have been established to support training and development work in specific countries. Cancer Relief India, a registered charity set up in 1990 by a British palliative care nurse, Gilly Burn, continues to provide specialist palliative care training to Indian doctors and nurses. The achievements of this small but prolific charity are far-reaching: the training of many doctors and nurses, which has enabled them to influence change in clinical practice and improvement in the quality of palliative care offered to patients, funding of several projects including a hospice and the first hospital-based palliative care team, funding of medical equipment and educational material, and, for the future, the development of an education center for people from all over India.

In Poland, a contributor to the development of their 160-strong hospice and palliative care services has been the UK charity, Polish Hospices Fund, which has again played a substantial role in funding training in palliative care and in the providing of an emergency cash fund, books, equipment, and supplies. Hospice development in Russia has been supported through the efforts of several individuals and also by a British charity, the British-Russian Hospice Society, which periodically sends out a small team of British-trained doctors and nurses to provide on-the-spot training courses. Resources are usually scarce, and everything has to be taught through interpreters, but the courses are generally extremely well received and highly evaluated.

On a more individual basis, a few overseas hospices are fortunate in being linked directly to a British-based charitable trust which has been set up specifically to support that particular hospice. A few hospices in Kenya, Uganda, Poland, and Romania benefit from such a relationship.

Hospice is now a worldwide philosophy and is active in six continents of the world. We are privileged that the Hospice Information Service at St. Christopher's has been able to play its role in the world of hospice care.

# 14

# The Ryder Italia Experience in Rome

**Giovanni Creton, M. D.**

Ryder Italia is a nonprofit organization for the home care of terminally ill cancer patients. It was set up as a branch of the Sue Ryder Foundation in November, 1984. Thanks to its social merits, Ryder Italia was officially recognized as a nonprofit organization by the president of the Italian Republic.

At present, Ryder Italia has a team of four doctors, six nurses, one social workers, and the necesssary administrative staff. In addition to the home care staff, there are a number of volunteers who are directly involved in patient care as well as in various fundraising activities.

The Ryder Italia staff currently provides care for 25–30 patients in their homes, visiting each patient daily. In its 10 years of activity it has cared for more than a terminally ill thousand cancer patients. More than 80% died in their home.

## ESTABLISHING A PALLIATIVE CARE PROGRAM IN ROME

The history of Ryder Italia reflects to some extent the development of cancer research and care in all Western countries.

In the early 1980s, special centers were being established for the treatment of neoplastic diseases in Rome, as well as in other parts of Italy. The first successful results achieved through chemotherapy and, especially, radiotherapy, enabled cancer patients to live longer. Both the patients and their doctors, however, were faced with the problem of the quality of life.

The high incidence of neoplastic disease and the high number of treatment failures led hospitals and public opinion to focus on the need to create teams not only for cure-oriented treatment, but also for the care of those patients—about 50% of the cases—for whom there is no cure.

The extent of this need can be gauged from the statistics. In Rome, in the 1980s, about 10,000 of this city's more than three million people died each year because of some disease. About six thousand of these deaths were attributable to cancer—and about 70% of these people died in hospitals because Rome had no suitable care centers.

There was also no home care for terminally ill cancer patients in Rome. The only type of home care available was limited to ill but self-sufficient elderly people. In other words, a person ill with a serious disease had no option other than going to a public or private hospital, and this is where most of the deaths occurred.

In the meantime, in the rest of Europe and in the United States, the first attempts were being made to care for terminally ill people on the basis of what is now called palliative care.

The Sue Ryder Foundation, famous all over the world for its help to people in need, decided in 1984 to establish a support program for cancer patients in Rome. The new program was intended to build on what other nations were already learning through their palliative care experiences. This initiative soon came up against the difficulties involved in translating the vision of a new type of health care program into practice. Nevertheless, the program has gone forward.

The combination of two groups of people made it possible to start a home-care program: a small number of oncologists, who felt the need to continue to care for their patients when they were in their terminal stage, and a few foreign nurses, who had had some experience of home care abroad. It was, in fact, a radiotherapist and a nurse who comprised the home care team during the home care program's first six months of operation.

The staff was gradually increased in the following months, utilizing funds from the Sue Ryder Foundation that could allow the program to function for the first 12–18 months. During the first years of its activity, Ryder Italia received extraordinarily generous support from the families of patients who were cared for by its medical and nursing team. Many of these families became the first true supporters of the program, and some are still strongly involved.

Public opinion welcomed the initiative; some doctors resisted it. These physicians did not believe it was possible to care for terminally ill patients in their homes. They contended that hospice care, the only modality familiar to them, was also the only acceptable approach. Over the first two or three years, the momentum to keep the home care program going was provided mainly by the families who had experienced the services of Ryder Italia. During this period of time hospitals mostly showed indifference, sometimes hostility, and only rarely interest and attention.

Another interesting factor in the first few years was the difference in the attitudes shown by medical and nursing staffs. Doctors did not seem able to regard patients as persons with their own individual requirements. Instead, they persisted in viewing them as patients to be treated. Nurses had a completely different perception. Seeing patients daily, the nurses were more accustomed to recognizing and attempting to meet all the needs of their patients, including the psychological.

The sensitivity expressed in the attitudes of the nursing staff has become a characteristic feature of the Ryder Italia team. To this day, the team has had greater ease in training nurses than doctors. It is not by chance that a decade after the beginning of its activity Ryder Italia has a team of professional nurses, most of whom have had some experience of home care in other nations.

The first years of our activity demonstrated how much people needed this service. At the time, however, the team was very small, and care was offered mainly to those patients whose families were willing to cooperate. The strong involvement of the family in the care of a dying patient allowed the team to see their psychological needs as well, and to seek the help of a psychologist who could meet those needs that are usually ignored in a hospital. All too often, hospitalized patients who are incurable are considered to be psychological burdens and left completely alone by the family who, in any case, would be with them only during visiting hours.

A main purpose of the Ryder Italia program in its early years was abolishing the ingrained practice of care of terminally ill people. Additionally, it was our purpose to allow and encourage the family to be with the patient in the last weeks of his/her life. The ongoing relationship between our team and the patient's family proved essential from a financial point of view as well. Ryder Italia offers its care services free of charge. Apart from the initial support from the Sue Ryder Foundation, the organization's economic survival has been made possible by donations.

Many who came into contact with our team during the early years decided to start working as volunteers. They suggested that we organize volunteer training courses for all those who wanted to help either with patient care, fundraising activities, or both.

As time went by, Ryder Italia became a major reference point for the home care of cancer patients in Rome. Not only did we provide direct care to more than a thousand patients in our first decade, but we have offered advice to another 300 people on how to relieve physical and psychological pain and the assistance of voluntary workers. Every day we respond to requests for these services.

# PROBLEMS OFTEN ENCOUNTERED BY PALLIATIVE CARE PROGRAMS

On the basis of the experience gathered so far, we can identify a number of problems which are probably encountered by other organizations offering the same type of care.

The first one is certainly the financial issue. This problem is experienced by all nonprofit organizations. The results achieved and the good quality of our service convinced other private philanthropies, such as the Shanker Foundation, and the Lefebvre Foundation, to support us with grants for our staff. Additionally, many volunteers raise funds through concerts, theater performances, bazaars, and jumble sales, and also publicize the association's purposes.

Another major difficulty we found was the lack of hospital beds for the last few days of a dying person's life. Some people could not be cared for adequately at home for physical or social reasons, and no hospital beds were available for this purpose. This was probably the worst problem that Ryder Italia had to face here in Rome, even though there are many hospitals operated by religious organizations. It has never been possible to secure their cooperation to hospitalize patients who are in the most difficult situations.

We therefore have had to resort to alternative solutions, such as the use of paid staff, or volunteers who are willing to spend the night with those patients who live alone and have expressed the wish to avoid the hospital and die at home.

This problem should not be underestimated. About five hundred thousand people over the age of 65 live in Rome. Half of these people live alone. If we consider those who are aged over 75, we see that there are a great many widows who live in economically difficult situations and without any family members who could help our home care team.

As time went by, our service developed and the demands placed on it increased. We decided to include a social worker in our team to evaluate all the problems linked with our home care services and with the families who request our help.

Data collected over the past three years indicate that more than 30% of the requests to Ryder Italia come from people who live alone or spend most of their time alone. These people, therefore, need more than just our home care service. A number of problems arise when these people are no longer self-sufficient and independent. Cooking meals and cleaning the house are among the most salient practical problems. No less important, though, is the feeling of loneliness that is likely to be experienced throughout the day.

## RESPONDING TO PROBLEMS

The experiences of Ryder Italia in its first decade show the need for continued development and innovation. An important example is our perception that the present trend advocating home care and the involvement of the whole family does not address the needs of all terminally ill cancer patients. We believe it is necessary to establish centers such as the Sue Ryder Homes or the hospices created in Anglo-Saxon countries.

The aging of Italy's population, especially in Rome, makes his goal a high priority. At present, the average household here is made up of 2.7 people. The average number of children per woman is 1.3. In the next few years we will witness an increase in the number of households made up of only one or two persons. It is therefore unrealistic to think that such small households could provide assistance in the home care of a terminally ill patient.

One of the most interesting aspects of our experience is that we had to create a completely new organization in a city that did not have any type of home care service for terminally ill cancer patients. We therefore aimed at three goals:

- Creating a care service that could meet the social, psychological, and health needs of the ill;
- Training staff for this type of care service, bearing in mind that medical and nursing schools still offer no courses in what is now called palliative care; and
- Overcoming the "cultural" problem concerning patients, their families, and the hospitals and/or social centers which theoretically should have taken care of these patients.

The only home care services in Rome were those provided by religious organizations, such as Caritas and Comunita di S. Egidio, with whom we still cooperate. However, these religious organizations tended to offer help mainly to the elderly, the homeless, and the ill who live alone, but they never tried to set up well-structured organizations for the larger spectrum of patients. On the contrary, Ryder Italia, considering all the real needs of a terminally ill patient cared for in his/her home, has tried to create a support system that can adjust to individual patients' needs and to interact with their specific social environments.

The role of volunteers became central as this goal was translated into action. The extraordinary willingness and skill of the volunteers enabled us to create an environment somehow similar to hospice in the patient's own home.

For example, one of the first patients cared for by Ryder Italia was an elderly lady who lived alone in Rome with no family. She had spent her whole life working as a volunteer in her neighborhood to help people in need. When our team started working with her, she was still functioning quite well, even though her cancer of the intestine had made her partially dependent on other people.

As weeks went by, her tumor worsened. She became totally dependent on other people as she could no longer prepare her meals. She told us she did not want to end up in a hospital, and we tried to find a way to manage her difficult situation. Ryder Italia was limited in experience and personnel resources at that time: we had a doctor, three nurses, and a few volunteers. Nevertheless, we tried to take turns so that somebody would always be with her.

This difficult experience motivated us to recruit and train volunteers who were willing to intervene in similar situations. These include cases of families with a terminally ill child when the parents are not able to cope, as well as the elderly person who is not self-sufficient, or any terminally ill cancer patient who lives alone.

Our volunteers are therefore a central element, especially in the most difficult situations, where the lack of a residential hospice or similar resource forces us to look for alternatives to a hospital admission. Most patients do not want to go to a hospital.

## MOVING AHEAD

The home care services offered by Ryder Italia for more than a decade have gradually changed in response to the needs expressed by the patients' families. At first we cared for patients with families that could help. This approach was in keeping with the small size of our staff: we had to rely on the help of the patient's family. As our staff increased, it became possible to care for other patients as well. At present, the requests for help we receive reflect the social composition of Rome's population—which is aging and has a high percentage of people living alone.

On the basis of the experiences gained in recent years, we have reached the conclusion that it is absolutely necessary to create something similar to a hospice. This facility could also be a center for the provision of home care services supported by a group of volunteers. Such a hospice could become a model for the future of health care services for the seriously ill and especially for the terminally ill.

We have noticed that people are asking for a different way of caring for the terminally ill. In the past, this task had been left to hospitals. Once in the hospital, terminally ill patients were left practically alone, with no palliative care. People are now asking for alternative care centers, where terminally ill people can spend their last days surrounded by qualified medical and nursing staff, as well as by people who are sensitive to their psychological and human needs.

Ryder Italia's experience was possible because Italy, along with other industrialized countries, is changing in many ways. These changes are affecting how people live and die. The family no longer can be assumed to be a resource capable of helping and supporting the elderly and the ill, although some such families still exist. The task must be taken over by new social structures which, by and large, have yet to be created. Even these structures will not be able to meet all the requirements of those who are ill or dying. This is why the role of voluntary workers is so important. Individuals who can no longer express their own feelings of solidarity within a traditional family still need and deserve the support of caring people. We must find a way to create a future society that can respond to the fundamental human needs of all its members. In this vital and challenging endeavor, palliative/hospice care has a major contribution to make.

## REFERENCES

Koren, M. J. (1986). Home care: Who cares? *New England Journal of Medicine, 314,* 917–920.

Smith, A. (1985). Hospice, the future. *British Medical Journal, 291,* 1670.

Spilling, R. (1986). *Terminal care at home.* Oxford: Oxford University Press.

Ward, A. (1982). Standards for home care services for the terminally-ill.*Community Medicine, 4,* 276–279.

# 15

# The Beginnings of Hospice Care Under Communist Regime: The Cracow Experience

Janina Jujawska Tenner, M. D.

On the 29th of September, 1981, the Society of Friends of the Sick, HOSPICJUM, was registered in Cracow, Poland. It was the first hospice society in Central and Eastern Europe, which at that time was under Communist regime.

Hospicjum is an independent charitable society which aims at "helping the terminally ill at the very end of their lives, giving them medical, psychological, social and spiritual support according to their real needs; giving a helping hand to their families; gathering people of goodwill prepared to take part in such activities" (Statut Towarzystwa Przyjaciol Chorych [HOSPICJUM], 1981). The Society is governed by a management council that is elected every three years by a general meeting of all the members. The management council consists of a president, vice president for medical affairs, vice president for hospice building affairs, secretary, treasurer, volunteer coordinator, and three others.

The Society works in the province of Cracow, which has a population of 1,230,000. There are nearly three thousand cancer deaths in this area every year.

## THE INITIAL PHASE

The registration of the Society ended the preparatory period that had started in the 1970s. The idea of building a hospice facility was born at that time among a group of parishioners of The Lord's Ark Church in Nowa Huta, the industrial district of Cracow. This group was composed mostly of ordinary citizens. They were employees of the big steel factories and their families. One physician was a member of the group. These parishioners were motivated by their Christian faith. They looked for a way to express their love and practice effective compassion for people in need.

Mrs. Halina Bortnowska, an outstanding philosopher and journalist engaged in the religious education of adults, influenced the group in the direction of care for very sick and dying people. There were also some other reasons for this decision. The initiators had had their own painful experiences with the National Health Service, which had no program to care for the dying. Families who wanted to help their terminally ill relatives in hospitals often were helpless to do so because they were not allowed on the wards.

At that time, some information about the hospice movement was starting to become available in Poland. A few books were published that proposed a more open attitude toward death and dying, as opposed to the prevailing silence and denial (Bortnowska, 1959; Kubler-Ross, 1979; Pearson, 1973).

The people who were thinking of establishing a hospice in Poland wanted to keep a custom that was derived from their rural culture. This custom compels people to keep their sick at home, to look after them, and to gather around their beds at the time of death. Unfortunately, the poor housing conditions in the industrial district made nursing the terminally ill at home very difficult. The hospice was meant to be a home rather than an institution. Families and friends were supposed to participate in nursing and other hospice activities on a voluntary basis.

The parishioners prepared themselves for this task by taking care of patients dying of cancer who had been admitted to the local hospital. The doctor in charge of one of the wards close to The Lord's Ark parish invited volunteers to assist the hospital staff. The hospice project started with this small but significant first step. The initiators already had the conception that the hospice eventually was to become a training center for care of the terminally ill that would foster the attitude of full respect for the human person. It was supposed to represent an outlook on life and death that was contrary to the ruling Communist doctrine, as well as to break the common stereotypes on how to deal with dying people.

The founding team contacted St. Christopher's Hospice. Dame Cicely Saunders visited Cracow in 1978 and met with The Lord's Ark group of parishioners. She also lectured in the Oncology Centre. For cancer doctors in Cracow, this was the first contact with the hospice movement and with modern pain relief methods.

These methods were not put into practice at that time. Nevertheless, Dr. Saunders' visit prepared the foundation for subsequent palliative care activities.

Communist authorities resisted the idea of setting up the hospice. These authorities were opposed to anything that was not within their complete control. Furthermore, the mass media did not inform the community about the hospice. At this point, the possibility of legalizing the future hospice seemed rather remote. One may doubt if the enthusiastic group of parishioners would have succeeded if it had not been for the outbreak of "Solidarity," the great independent movement, in 1980 and 1981. This movement weakened the governing power, thereby opening some opportunities for new developments.

A few stories about the hospice movement started to appear in the local newspapers, and the initiators were able to send invitations to other people who might be interested in this project. The replies included some from physicians from the Oncology Centre. They remembered Dame Cicely's lecture and were convinced of the importance of changing attitudes toward dying people. The project also received the support of the local "Solidarity" union. When the original team became larger and stronger, the decision was made to set up an open secular organization. After many further delays and difficulties, "The Society of the Friends of the Sick HOSPICJUM in Cracow" was duly registered as a charity association.

## THE EARLY PHASE

The Society started its official work in 1981. At that time, the focus was to build up the awareness of the members and to promulgate the idea that proper hospice care could improve a cancer patient's quality of life even when the disease was incurable. In addition, the Society intended to train volunteers, implement home care, raise funds, and erect a freestanding hospice.

The educational component of our mission was difficult to perform. There had been a long period of time when cultural changes, together with the totalitarian regime, had banished death and dying from social consciousness. In Poland, this process had probably been accomplished more efficiently than in Western countries. The total control of scientific life did not help research on death and dying. The words themselves were avoided because they elicited fear and anxiety.

The unwillingness and inability to discuss death had become such a problem that at one of the general meetings in the 1980s it was suggested that the Society should talk about care for chronically ill patients—and not mention "dying," because this word would scare people and make it difficult to recruit volunteers. This opinion on the part of the public was shared by many health care professionals. It was their belief that pain was inseparable from dying of cancer. Morphine was given to dying patients only in their last days of life. This practice was justified as a measure to prevent dying people from becoming addicts.

A political problem further complicated the situation. The government introduced martial law in the early 1980s, resulting in a temporary severing of links between Poland and Western countries. Professional literature did not reach Poland. Personal contacts were interrupted. For example, the author of this chapter was refused a passport to visit St. Christopher's Hospice in 1982. This interference with the communication process increased the intellectual and emotional demands on members of the Society and also caused some errors.

Nevertheless, the hospice project continued to develop. Training of volunteers started in 1983. These training courses are intended for nonprofessionals and have since been offered on an annual basis. The first patients were given systematic home care in 1984. This service was provided by nonprofessional volunteers and by physicians and nurses who donated their time and effort.

## The First Patient

The first patient who was treated according to the World Health Organization guidelines of pain control was a man of 61 with recurrent rectal cancer. His sacral bone had been destroyed and replaced by a huge tumor that prevented the patient from lying on his back. He had a colostomy and an indwelling catheter. His general condition was relatively good, but he suffered from incapacitating pain.

No one listened to him carefully and no one tried to speak to him. As a consequence of his social isolation as well as his physical condition, the patient was taking a lot of drugs, nearly the whole spectrum of available painkillers (with the exception of morphine). These drugs were taken in uncontrolled doses and in a chaotic way. This undisciplined use of drugs did not alleviate the pain effectively and caused severe side effects. On the first home visit, the hospice doctor found the muddled patient lying in a fetal position on the floor and crying from pain. His terrified wife was sitting behind him in great despair.

The pain was brought under control after the physician took away most of the previous medicines and prescribed oral morphine every four hours with the adjuvant drugs. The patient remained under hospice care until his death nine months later. The local doctor had limited knowledge of pain control, but was willing to cooperate. The family was also ready to help. With this new pattern of support, it was possible to alleviate the other problems connected with the progressing disease, and the home was put in order and at peace again.

The family was taught how to look after the patient. His son equipped the flat with handrails. This gave the patient some independence as long as he was able to talk. When the patient later became bedridden, an antipressure mattress was delivered to provide more comfort. With his pain now controlled, the man was able to read, watch television, and enjoy his grandchildren and friends. He spoke openly to his doctor about his illness. He had accepted the nearness of death, but at the same time was willing to make the best of his remaining life. No longer ravaged by pain, the patient had the opportunity and strength to put all his affairs in order before he died.

## Establishing the Hospice Facility: Coins in a Basket

By 1984 the Society had raised enough money to start construction of a hospice facility. The building was to be situated on a plot close to The Lord's Ark church. This piece of land had been given to the Society by the local authorities in 1981.

The city council now stopped the project from continuing. There had been protests from some people who lived in the vicinity of the proposed hospice. They claimed that the area was already overcrowded, that the building would threaten the environment, and that the hospice itself would hurt their feelings.

The authorities justified their attitude by adding that the National Health Service could provide proper care for everybody who needs it. The idea of hospice was denounced as foreign to the Polish tradition that impending death should not be disclosed and discussed with patients because this acknowledgement of reality would destroy the patient's hope (HOSPICJUM, 1985a, 1985b; Konarski, 1985).

One can suppose that the political powers hostile to any independent activities were responsible for instigating and supporting this opposition. However, there was also ignorance; the real fear of death, and the unwillingness to change the pervasive stereotypical approach to death. As time passed and the ruling Communist system became weaker and weaker, it became possible to argue with these opinions in the local and national media. Friendly journalists took advantage of this opportunity. Therefore, in spite of the authorities' effort, the hospice idea became well-known and was welcomed by the majority of the public.

The people of Nowa Huta also accepted the hospice. On one Sunday morning in February, 1989, the parishioners attending Mass in The Lord's Ark church were asked to drop a single coin into a basket while passing the doorway. This action would be a sign of approving the hospice project. On this day 11,000 coins were collected—meaning that 37% of the citizens approved of having the hospice facility in their area.

Meanwhile, the Society bought a small house which has been serving as its abode ever since. Above all, however, the Society was trying to reverse the authorities' 1984 decision which forbade the construction of a freestanding hospice. There were several court hearings and, finally, in 1989, the Supreme Administrative Court decided that the freestanding hospice could be built on the Society's plot in Nowa Huta. That year marked the fall of the Communist system as well as a new period in the Society's development. The Society's activities no longer were hindered by prejudiced bureaucrats. There were only the "normal" obstacles ahead.

## THE GROWING PHASE

The Society started to erect a freestanding hospice in 1989. On May 4, 1991, the cornerstone was laid for the future St. Lazarus Hospice. This is to be a full spectrum center of palliative care with the best possible standard of service, modelled on St. Christopher's Hospice in London. There will be an inpatient unit with 35 beds, an outpatient clinic with home care service, a day care center, social department, bereavement services, and educational center with library and lecture hall. The building is already finished and the interior decorating work is presently being carried on. The formal opening of the Hospice has been planned for 1996.

The completion and opening of St. Lazarus Hospice is dependent on the Society's funds. The funding sources include members' fees, fundraising activities, and donations from private persons and institutions in Poland and abroad. For the last 2 years, the building project has also been supported by the City Council.

There were some difficult times when the Society was short of money, but the construction work, even if it sometimes had to slow down, never stopped. The Society has many friends throughout the country and abroad who support its work. Among them are an anonymous sponsor from the United Kingdom who was informed about the Society's needs by Dame Cicely Saunders. Other sponsors include The Krakow Hospice Education Fund and the Polish Hospices Fund of the United Kingdom, the Knights of St. Lazarus Order from Vienna, The Friends of Hospicium and Koch's Foundation in the USA, The Royal Society of Friends of Rose, and The Friends of the Polish Hospice in Belgium.

Additionally, the Polish foundation "Help Cracow's Hospice" was set up on the initiative of the Society's management council to earn money for construction and maintenance. The foundation runs shops with medical supplies and sells publications about palliative care. It is thought that in the future the St. Lazarus Hospice will be maintained partly by funds of the Society and those of the local foundation, and partly by contracts with the National Health Service.

In the 1990s the Outpatients' Pain Control and Palliative Care Clinic and Home Care Service was established with a paid professional team of physicians and nurses. Together with the voluntary workers, they are looking after about 300 patients yearly. Besides pain and symptom control, the home team provides psychological, social, and emotional support to dying people and their families. Financially needy patients are also supplied with necessary medical utensils.

The Society could not exist without its volunteers. They give their time, skill, and commitment to the dying people. About 50 nonprofessional but trained volunteers are participating in home care. Another group helps to run the Society. The other volunteers organize the Society's activities, perform office work, supervise the construction of the building, raise funds, provide training for health care workers and volunteers, take part in public education, run a professional library, provide transport and accommodation for the Society's guests, and take care of the Society's house and its garden. Future volunteers are found through personal contact with the Society's activities and through articles in the media.

The Society places great importance on the continuous education of its members and the public. Professional personnel are trained at St. Christopher's Hospice. "Help Cracow's Hospice" has translated and published two WHO booklets on pain relief and palliative care. The Society has participated in preparing another booklet on cancer pain treatment under the editorship of the Ministry of Health. This booklet has been distributed among physicians and nurses in Poland. Additionally, members of the Society initiate and take part in many educational projects for health care workers and medical and nursing students in the area. The Society also inspires the mass media to inform the public that people dying of cancer have the right to obtain effective palliative care and be free from pain.

## HOSPICE CARE IN OTHER PARTS OF POLAND

In other parts of Poland, specialized and comprehensive care for people in the terminal stages of progressive disease is carried out in two ways: by nongovernmental organizations (e.g., the hospices) and by the National Health Service.

After the hospice movement was introduced in Cracow, programs were established in Gdansk (Hospicium Pallotinum, 1984) and Poznan (St. John Kanty Hospicium, 1985). Later, additional units were organized throughout Poland, mostly in connection with local parishes. Hospice Forum, an umbrella organization, now has a membership of 48 local hospice programs. The Forum files indicate that some hospices are independent, some partially financed by Church charities, and some by state authorities. Together they look after about 1,200 patients monthly, predominantely in home care. However, there are also 12 hospice residential facilities and six day care centers. As of 1994, there were nearly 900 professional and nonprofessional volunteers working in Polish hospices, along with 236 paid professional employees.

In addition, palliative care on a larger scale has been provided by the National Health Service under the guidance of Prof. Jacek Luczak, who set up the Palliative Care Department of the School of Medicine in Poznan in 1991. This Department also conducts educational, research, and policy-planning activities on a national scale. There is close operation between Cracow Hospice and the Palliative Care Department in Poznan.

## SUCCESSES, FAILURE, AND CHALLENGES

A positive change in the public attitude toward setting up hospices has made itself known in just the past few years. The general opinion is now in favor of hospice.

There is still a lot of personal resistance toward the hospice idea among many health care workers and the general public. Some doctors do not trust the WHO methods of pain control and/or are reluctant to communicate honestly with the dying.

A few former opponents of hospice have expressed their past and current thinking with me. The former chief of the National Health Service in Cracow Province, now retired, told me that he did believe in those days that the NHS could meet all the medical and social needs of the people. He cited his order that patients should not be allowed to die on the hospital corridors, where they were usually placed to save the better beds in the rooms for those who could be cured. During the 1970s and 1980s, though, he could not accept the open attitude toward death that was being encouraged by hospice, and was also suspicious of the Church. He assured me, however, that he had had nothing to do with the protest of the neighbors against building the hospice. Now this retired physician has changed his mind because times have changed. Presently, he is convinced that there is a need for specialized care of dying people.

A former lecturer in sociology in one of the high schools was the leader of the neighbors' protest. She has not changed her mind. She remains an opponent of hospice residential facilities. There have been no qualms of conscience regarding her previous opposition against us. She has not admitted that this opposition was inspired by the Communist authorities at the time.

Contrast this with the attitude of another previous opponent. This woman is director of a gastronomy school next door to St. Lazarus. She has become one of our supporters, allowing us to use the school facilities free for our meetings, and her storeroom for our goods. She also encourages her students to do voluntary work for the hospice.

Resistance does not come only from some professional health care personnel and members of the general public. There are also some patients who cannot handle the thought of approaching death which they link with hospice care. These people do not ask for help in time and therefore suffer unnecessarily. A long-term comprehensive program of education for both professionals and public should therefore be developed and made available on a consistent basis. There is also an urgent need for a system of evaluating the effectiveness of the palliative care program's implementation. These are among the challenges.

The Society of Friends of the Sick HOSPICJUM in Cracow is now 15 years old. This period of time provides the opportunity for reflection on successes and failures.

Starting with the mistakes, one now can see that in the 1970s and early 1980s the founding members were very enthusiastic, but rather naive, and lacking experience in palliative care. This combination led to the expensive and perhaps ostentatious project of constructing a hospice facility. A simpler and cheaper building probably would have been finished by now. There was also an overestimation of the potential of voluntary service in providing home care. One cannot ensure competent and consistent care for more than a very few dying patients by relying heavily on caregivers who can offer their services only after completing their daily duties and who cannot prescribe drugs. The professional service should therefore have been started earlier.

Initiating and implementing home care for cancer patients in Cracow can be regarded as a great accomplishment of the Society. Its main success, however, lies in introducing the idea of hospice care for terminally ill people in Poland. The struggle with the regime for permission to build the hospice made the hospice movement famous and impressed itself on the public consciousness. It also gave rise to many other such projects all over the country and, later, to the inclusion of palliative care in the structure of the National Health Service. There are now palliative care programs and grassroots hospice programs throughout much of the nation.

# REFERENCES

Bortnowska, H. (Ed.) (1959). *Sens choroby, sens zycia, sns smierci.* Znak: Krakow.
Konarski, L. (1985). Umrzec wsrod ludzi. *Przeglad Tygodniowy, 36,* 5.
Kubler-Ross, E. (1979). *Rozmowy o smierci i umieraniu.* Warsaw: Pax.
Pearson, L. (Ed.) (1973). Postepowanie z czlowiekiem umierajacym PWN: Warsaw.
Statut Towarzystwa Przyjaciol Chorych HOSPICJUM. (1981). Krakow.

# 16

# The Russian Approach to Hospice Care

**Virginia-Ann Gumley**

---

> *One cannot understand Russia with the mind alone.*
> *She cannot be measured with an ordinary yardstick.*
> *She is unique and stands alone—*
> *One can only believe in Russia.*
> Fyodor Tyutechev (1803–1973)

As I attempt to outline the Russian approach to hospice care, these words have taken on a new meaning, and I hope that as this story unfolds you, too, will agree with the poet's words. The account I offer here is drawn from my personal experience since 1991 and information given to me by my Russian colleagues.

## INTRODUCTION

The development of hospice care in Russia should be seen within the social context of the Russian health care system and medical education.

The growth of hospice care in Russia has been quite phenomenal since the first hospice opened in St. Petersburg in 1990. It would be impossible to give an exact accounting of the number of hospice programs that have already achieved some level of operation. However, it can be said that there are programs developing now in at least 15 regions, some having several programs underway. This activity is particularly strong in St. Petersburg, which has six programs, including hospices, palliative care units, and home care teams. It is difficult to grasp the rapidity of growth of hospice programs in Russia since the collapse of the Soviet Union. This growth has occurred despite political turmoil, social upheaval, and economic stringency.

The scope of this chapter will be confined to Russia. There are embryonic developments in some of the republics, but it has proved difficult to obtain detailed and reliable information. In Russia there is a very good network of communication among oncologists which may, in part, explain the growth of hospice care. For the most part, hospice development has been limited to care for people with advanced cancer.

Telyukov (1991) writes that "Soviet reformers were striving to reconstruct a health care system plagued by chronic underfunding, antiquated and deteriorating facilities, inadequate supplies, outmoded equipment, poor morale, and few incentives for health care workers." According to Telyukov's report, the Russian health care system has a great many hospital beds and a large system of polyclinics. These are staffed by a very high number of physicians. Educational preparation is divided into medical student education, which takes place in a university setting, and middle medical professional education. The former program is for physicians; the latter program is for nurses and *feldshers* (primary medical caregivers). The physicians and other medical staff receive low salaries and occupy a relatively low-status niche in society. WHO statistics present a troubled picture of the health of the Russian people. Life expectancy has been declining rather than rising. Suicide has joined heart disease and cancer as the top killers.

## THE BEGINNINGS OF HOSPICE CARE IN RUSSIA

There appear to have been two separate although simutaneous threads of development which now are coming together. The first pain control department was established in Moscow in 1987. Four years later, legislation was passed to regulate the prescribing of pain medication (Novokov, 1995). In 1993, an expert committee was formed to organize palliative care for inoperable cancer patients. This committee provided the impetus to organize the first palliative care conference in Moldova in 1993. Three models of palliative care delivery are now developing: pain control departments, hospice units, and palliative care units, each with a home care service (Bryuzgin, 1991).

The recent revival of a pre-Bolshevik nursing order in Moscow reveals that some female members of the Tsar's family were also much involved in a sisterhood concerned with bringing care to those who were dying. Emphasis often was on soldiers, particularly during the Crimean War. This nursing order now focuses upon bringing care and comfort to dying people in the general population.

Another thread of development has been associated with the work of Victor Zorza, a former journalist of Polish-Russian origins. The first modern hospice in Russia opened in St. Petersburg in 1990 as a result of Zorza's inspiration. His only daughter died of cancer in the mid-1970s in an English hospice. He was so impressed with the care she received and the way in which she died that he set himself the task of establishing similar services for the Russian people. Zorza spread the hospice idea in Russia through radio and television interviews and newspaper articles. His influential book, *A Way to Die: Living to the End,* was published first in English (1981), and a decade later in Russian.

The first St. Petersburg hospice is now a well established 30-bed inpatient unit with a home care team. It is situated to the north of the city. It is funded in part by the health care system and in part by a charitable organization in the United Kingdom.

Shortly after the establishment of the St. Petersburg hospice service, a course was offered for physicians interested in palliative care. This proved to be the beginning of a concentrated education and training program for health professions. Zorza gained the support of medical professionals in the United Kingdom in organizing and implementing this course. He planned to organize a similar course in Moscow for nurses, but was unable to find nurses who were willing or able to go to Moscow for the prolonged period he had envisaged.

His desperation was at its peak when he attended St. Christopher's Hospice International Conference in 1991 and made impassioned pleas for help for Russia. These pleas reached my ears by the end of the conference, and, with the support of the senior chaplain at St. Christopher's, I contacted Zorza to offer my services. I went to Moscow later that year along with several others, and we organized and implemented a course for nurses in palliative care (Gumley, 1992). In retrospect, it can be seen that these two courses had a catalytic effect on hospice development throughout Russia.

Since the establishment of the first hospice in St. Petersburg, there have been various creative ways in which the development has proceeded. Most of these methods have come about because of the lack of finances. One organization in the United Kingdom that has contributed much to this development is Charity Know How, an initiative of the British, Foreign, and Commonwealth Office. Its aim is to finance and promote the concept of partnership development in the voluntary sector in Eastern Europe and Russia. For example, town-twinnings exist between Yaroslavl and Exeter, and between Perm and Oxfordshire County. Partnerships of this kind have helped to develop and finance hospices in Russia. Moscow hospice development has benefitted from Victor Zorza's iniative and from the British-Russian Hospice society, of which he is the chairman. All the St. Petersburg programs have benefitted from the St. Petersburg Health Care Trust, a charitable organization based in the United Kingdom.

Many subsequent courses have been given in other areas, including Omsk and Kemerova in Siberia. There are also plans to develop hospice care in the Chelyabinsk region to be supported by Aid to Russian Christians, another United Kingdom-based charitable organization.

The "August coup" took place not long after the course in Moscow had been given. There was silence from the palliative care people in Russia. Early in 1992, however, I received the good news that the second hospice in the Tula Region had just opened. This dramatic event came about as a result of the motivation and inspiration of Dr. Elmira Karajaeva, who had attended the first course for doctors in St. Petersburg, and some of her senior nurses, who had attended the course in Moscow. With this news came the invitation for me to go to Tula. Almost at the same time, an invitation arrived for me to go to Ulyanovak to undertake some teaching. With the financial support of Charity Know How, I was able to return to Russia. Since that time, all my expenses have been covered by Charity Know How, and this has ensured the continued developments. After 1992, so many invitations were received to teach in Russia that it became apparent to me that I could not keep up with the demand. I decided to concentrate on one or two regions and attempt to build a networking system through which the Russians would be able to help themselves by sharing information and skills.

I chose to concentrate my efforts outside Moscow and St. Petersburg as it seemed, according to reports, that the majority of external support was going to these two cities, and that other regions were keen to develop their own hospice care services. My guiding principle was to go only where I was invited and to enable partnerships to develop.

## DEVELOPMENTS IN THE TULA REGION

The Lomintsevesky Hospice was the second to open. It is a 30-bed inpatient unit that is situated in a small village on the outskirts of Tula City. Tula is largely a coal-mining area that is south of Moscow and on the outer perimeters of the Chernobyl incident.

It has been reported that the incidence of cancer is rising here, particularly thyroid and lung cancers. The inpatient unit is financed chiefly by an American organization. The hospice program is within the state health care system and financed by the regional budget. The Regional Health Administration is sensitive to hospice development and provides support within the limits of its budget. The first 18 months of hospice development in Lomintsevsky have been described by Karajaeva (1994). Four years after its establishment, Lomintsevesky Hospice appeared to be secure and has been described in one of the leading medical journals (Karajaeva, 1995). There are plans to develop a home care team working between the hospice and the oncology dispensary in Tula. Lack of finances remains a stumbling block to further developments at present. Another major problem is to obtain a constant supply of medications. This problem is encountered in all Russian hospices.

Lomintsevsky Hospice also enjoys a special "twinning relationship" with a London Church Sunday School. In 1993 the hospice was adopted by St. Mark's Church, Regent's Park Sunday School, who have undertaken to write twice a year and to send small gifts for patients and staff. This generosity has been mutual. Recently, a package arrived at St. Mark's which contained pictures made by the local school children in the kindergarten and primary school classes from Lomintsevesky. This local school supports the hospice and visits the patients, so it seems to be important that they, too, can gain support by writing to St. Mark's Church Sunday School children.

The philosophy of hospice care is based on the World Health Organization's *Principles of Hospice Care*. This booklet and other relevant publications were translated into Russian (Bick, Chupiatova, & Gumley, 1994; Frampton & Twycross, 1994). These publications are now easily accessible in Russia.

## DEVELOPMENTS IN THE TYJUMEN REGION

The Tyjumen Region in Western Siberia is a large area with well-developed oil and gas industries. My contact with caregivers here came about unexpectedly. In October of 1993, the European School of Oncology (Moscow) planned a conference on cancer pain and palliative care in Kishinov, Moldova. I was invited to speak at this conference to meet with the many professionals who were interested in developing hospice care. One person who particularly impressed me with his enthusiasism and motivation was a young physician, Pavel Zotov. He shared his hopes for hospice development in Tyjumen and invited me to give a series of lectures there.

Some time passed before this trip could be arranged, and again it was financed by Charity Know How. When I arrived in Ryjumen on a sunny summer day and was met by Dr. Zotov, I was overwhelmed to learn of the developments that had taken place in the intervening nine months. A 10-bed anti-pain department had been established within the Regional Oncology Center which has both inpatient and outpatient facilities (Gumley, 1994).

Dr. Zotov is an anesthesist who has pioneered many new techniques in pain control, utilizing not only traditional methods, but also psychological approaches, such as relaxation and visual imagery. The anti-pain department has been very well received. It uses a multiprofessional team approach and has been holding seminars within the Regional Oncology Center for all health care professionals.

Other developments within Tyjumen include a 20-bed hospice inpatient unit financed from the city health budget and a home care service. Dr. Zotow has continued to play a leading role, not only in Tyjumen, but later in 1995, when he accompanied me to Ulyanovsk and assisted in teaching hospice personnel.

## DEVELOPMENTS IN THE ULYANOVSK REGION

The Ulyanovsk Region is represented in the radical democratic press as an "island of Communism" because of its low cost of living and provision of subsidized food. It is situated in hilly land on both sides of the middle stretch of the Volga River and has a reasonably healthy economy. The region has a population of approximately 1.4 million, most of whom live in the three major towns of Ulyanovsk, Dimitrovgrad, and Novoulyanovsk. Its industrial enterprises include a car plant and an aircraft plant. There is fertile agricultural land which enables the area to maintain a certain amount of self-sufficiency. This area was the birthplace of Lenin, and his legacies remain and influence all aspects of life in Ulyanovsk (Russia Briefing, 1995).

Ulyanovsk is taking a systematic, coherent, and logical approach to the development of palliative care services. I received an invitation to teach in Ulyanovsk in 1992, and the partnership has continued to develop. At the beginning it was a "triumvirate" relationship on the Russian side, with the three partners being the Ulyanovsk Branch Medical Faculty of Moscow State University, the Regional Oncology Dispensary, and the Regional Health Administration. A strategy for developing hospice services was established with the assistance of the WHO's Palliative Care Department in Geneva. There are yearly reviews to evaluate the progress.

The first stage of the strategy highlighted the need for various key personnel to become members of the European Association of Palliative Care and to subscribe to their philosophical approach. Also included was the identification of key personnel to visit other hospice units in Russia and to attend an international conference on palliative care.

The second stage of the strategy identified the Regional Plan for the Development of Hospice/Palliative Care in the Ulyanovsk Region. This plan was intended to ensure that a home care team would cover every part of the region, with an inpatient unit situated in both of the two major cities.

In December, 1994, the first home care team began its work. Several more home care programs quickly followed. There are now eight operational teams, each with transportation and each operating from the Ulyanovsk base. The inpatient building has been allocated with plans to open the first 10-bed unit in the near future. A small day care center started in 1994 and can accommodate four patients per day. In Dimitrovgrad, the home care service started in 1995, and was quickly followed by the opening of a five-bed in-patient unit. The chief doctors in both cities have been appointed and will be taking the developments forward, guided by the regional strategy. The local health administration has been fully supportive of these developments and has built provisions for palliative care into the budget agenda (Biktimirov, Bezvoritnye, & Gumley, 1994).

Two other major goals have been achieved. A curriculum has been devised and implemented for undergraduate medical students who now have the option of spending an elective period working alongside the hospice home care teams. A similar curriculum has been designed for *feldshers* and nurses and will soon be implemented in the medical college.

The final target for the second stage of the strategy was the foundation of an Association for Palliative Care in Ulyanovsk. This association was registered as a nongovernmental organization and a president appointed late in 1995. Its next step is to establish goals for the future.

The development of hospice care programs in the Ulyanovsk Region has been meticulous. The aim is to become the first such program in Russia to achieve WHO Collaborating Center Status. Intensive education has taken place in various hospitals throughout the area, including the Regional Oncology Center. Many television and radio programs have also been presented to educate the public about hospice. These programs have had the effect of creating a critical mass of public opinion that supports hospice development for Ulyanovsk.

The current developmental plan has taken a major step forward to embrace new partners, both in the United Kingdom and Ulyanovsk. Funding responsibility, administrative support, and management will be moved to Health Prom UK, an organization with experience in securing financial aid from United Kingdom and European bodies. It is hoped this arrangement will provide support for broader developments of hospice care. Several other organizations have either already contributed or stated that they wished to be involved. These include Medical Help for Russia, which has a successful track record of supplying humanitarian aid in response to requests. The Ulyanovsk region has requested equipment such as beds, bedside lockers, and wheelchairs to equip the hospice in Dimitrovgrad. Transportation has been supplied through a joint venture between a Ulyanovsk air freight organization with a base in the United Kingdom. East European Partnership, an initiative of Voluntary Services Overseas (UK), is providing and supporting a palliative care nurse from the UK to work alongside the emerging hospice teams.

Along the way, throughout all of these developments, many exciting events happened. For example, the Volga Brass Quintet, a section of the Ulyanovsk Philharmonic Orchestra, toured England at the invitation of the Cambridge University Musical Society. They visited St. Christopher's Hospice and generously gave a concert for patients and staff. They also gave a concert at St. Mark's Church, Regent's Park, an event that lead to the twinning arrangement between the church and the Lomintsevesky Hospice. The Volga Brass Quintet have also given concerts in Ulyanovsk in aid of hospice development.

## REAL-LIFE STORIES: PATIENTS AND THEIR FAMILIES

The rapid development of palliative care programs in Russia is admirable, but the essence of this movement lies with the patients and their families. As already mentioned, the Soviet health care system was suffering from chronic under-funding. Many health professionals were feeling powerless to carry out their responsibilities. Cancer care treatments were all focused on the acute and curative stage of the disease, with very limited resources for ongoing supportive care. The aim was to keep hospital bed occupancy at 100%. In consequence, the majority of patients spent long periods in the hospital, usually at regional centers.

The distance to travel to the regional center was often so great that many families were separated. At the time of diagnosis, many patients were already in the advanced stage of the disease and were sent home following radical treat-ments. Unfortunately, no adequate home support system existed. All too often, this sequence meant going home to die as a burden to their families. Additionally, it often meant going home to die without adequate pain medication. Many professionals felt uncomfortable with this situation, but also felt powerless to change the system. Hospitals achieved their ratings according to bed occupancy and discharge rate, not the quality of care for terminally ill patients and their families.

I have been told that many doctors and nurses used their own off-duty time to keep in touch with their ex-patients and to offer whatever little support they could. Clearly, the situation was very unsatisfactory for patients, families, and professional health care providers.

Hospice care for Russia was an idea whose time had come. I believe it was because of this "ripeness" that the hospice care philosophy spread so rapidly. The Russians were eager to find some solution to their situation and to be part of that solution. The "hospice idea" simply caught the imagination of the Russian people. The present system attempts to provide a comprehensive service for all cancer patients. Treatment for the cancer is received as the regional center. Followup treatment is provided at the polyclinic in their home towns. When the patient's disease advances he or she is introduced to the hospice service. Here are three brief real-life examples of the new hospice care approach in Russia.

## Grachev

*Age:*            22, a war veteran
*Diagnosis:*      Brain tumor, fourth stage

*Social History:* Single. Lives with his parents and older brother in a small flat on a high-rise block on the 12th floor.

*Background:*

Both parents are very hard working and deeply attached to their sons. The elder son, also a war veteran, has had alcohol-related problems since his return to civilian life, and has caused his parents very anxious times.

Grachev was a healthy young man up to 6 months ago, but began complaining of headaches and then had a series of epileptic fits. He was seen by a doctor in the polyclinic who referred him to the regional hospital, where he was diagnosed with a brain tumor. He had radical surgery and radiotherapy. Following an intensive period of rehabilitation, he was discharged home to the care of his parents. The surgery left him with residual left-sided weakness in both his arm and leg.

Over the next few months, the sight in his left eye gradually deteriorated. His mother attempted to get him referred back to the regional hospital, but was unsuccessful in doing so.

## Hospice Intervention

The hospice team was contacted and made an assessment visit. The assessment highlighted the fact that the mother was coping very well with Grachev, but that the father found it it difficult. The father had to work long hours to earn enough money to ensure sufficient medication for Grachev, and was out of the home for very long periods. The older son increased his alcohol consumption and was also absent from the home.

The hospice team decided to visit on a daily basis and did so for the final six weeks of Grachev's life. As his condition deteriorated, all nursing interventions were required, along with pain and symptom management. Emotional support was offered to the mother, and she knew she could contact the team at any time. Meanwhile, the team worried about breaking the bad news about Grachev's condition to the mother. They spent many hours in discussion amongst themselves, deciding to talk first to the mother and then try to talk to both parents together.

On the appointed day, the doctor and the nurse were about to commence their informational discussion—but the mother spoke first. "Before you say anything, I want to show you something." She brought everybody into another room, where she opened a cupboard and took out a man's suit. "This," she said, "is Grachev's burial suit! I bought it a month ago."

There was a lot of crying and shedding of tears at this moment. Later in the day, the team was able to have a discussion with both parents regarding Grachev's condition and his impending death.

Grachev died four days later. The team attended his funeral and have made a bereavement visit to the family. The psychologist will continue to be available to the family if required. (A bereavement service is now in its embryonic stage.)

# Irina

Age:              24
Diagnosis:        Ovarian tumor, pelvic and spinal secondaries
Social History:   Single, homeless, with a nine-year-old boy
Background:

Irina's parents died when she was 10 years old. She was brought up by her older sister. At the age of 15, Irina became pregnant, and was put out of her home. Little is known of what happened to her for the next few years. When her son was three years old, they both found shelter in the cloakroom of a school, where the teachers kept their presence secret. The teachers supported her with food and clothing over the next six years. It was one of the teachers who observed that her health was poor and, through a personal contact, persuaded a doctor to vist her. Irina was admitted to a hospital after the examination. Consultation took place among the medical staff. It was decided to contact one of their former colleagues who was now a hospice physician.

## Hospice Intervention

The hospice doctor met Irina and decided to offer her an inpatient bed. On admission Irina was a very thin, frail young woman with advanced ovarian cancer with pelvic ascites and partial cord compression. She was given a single room and the boy was also admitted with her. Irina settled in well and was liked by all the staff.

At this point she had several major problems. Irina was unable to move her legs and had retention of urine and bowel problems. Severe ascites caused her difficulties in breathing. The hospice staff was able to manage all these problems efficiently.

The more difficult problems for the hospice staff were how to enable Irina to face her advanced disease and make provisions for her son. They found it extremely difficult to talk openly with Irina regarding her prognosis. They also felt that she had had a miserable life and it just was not fair to inflict further pain. The team did decide, however to talk with her about her advancing disease, and to use the boy's future as the impetus for this conversation. The hospice staff arranged for the boy to go to summer camp, an event which Irina was thoroughly proud about. The boy enjoyed himself very much and will be starting school at the beginning of the next school year.

This story has not yet ended, but it illustrates the caring, compassionate, and humane approach that is embodied in hospice care.

## Vladimir

*Age:*               65
*Diagnosis:*         Small cell cancer of the lung
*Social History:*

Vladimir has been married for 40 years. He and his wife live in a well-maintained flat. Vladimir was an Air Force pilot and retired 10 years ago. He was diagnosed with lung cancer nine months ago. Vladimir had radical surgery (left lobectomy) followed by three courses of chemotherapy. He made a good recovery and returned home. Since his return home, he has visited the local polyclinic on a monthly basis and had a home assessment visit from the hospice team.

## Hospice Intervention

The hospice team described their service and explained what was available. Vladimir and his wife were very accepting of the hospice team and good relationships were formed. The hospice team visited once every two weeks. Vladimir has no problems at present, apart from shortness of breath.

His wife is extremely anxious about him, however, and the hospice team has identified that she will need ongoing support. The team has established a good relationship with her, which provides a sound basis for the future when they will be required in a more active role.

## CONCLUSION

The story has been told. Hospice/palliative care is now established in Russia. The spadework has been done by very many people, bringing together their various talents, skills, and attributes. However, the 1%, the final spark, is a gift. It is the indefinable "something" that has lifted a performance out of the ordinary; like a current released by a touch of a switch that lights a city, it illuminates the whole enterprise.

Today, with the vanishing of the old structures in Russia, many continue to hold on to their dreams of the past. One should therefore tread softly, not just out of courtesy or expediency, but out of respect.

In Russia, as you leave the big cities behind and travel on a few kilometers, you find that the road you encounter is not always smooth. In fact, large potholes appear. In the same way, difficulties were encountered by hospice pioneers within a health care system that had been starved of resources for decades. Few people have opposed the hospice movement, and these soon disappeared from sight when the conversation started to turn to the care of dying people. Much public and professional education remains to be done: this will be the mission of the leaders of tomorrow, as they carry the hospice idea forward.

# REFERENCES

Bick, M., KLChupiatova, V., & Gumley, V. (Eds.) (1994). *The principles and philosophy of hospice/palliative care.* London: Charity Know How.

Biktimirov, T., Bezvoritnye, V., & Gumley, V. (1994). *A programme of palliative care development in the Ulyanovsk Region.* Ulyanovsk: Moscow State University.

Bryuzgin, V. (1991). Pain and palliative care for cancer patients in the USSR. *Journal of Pain and Symptom Management, 6,* 1–2.

Frampton, D., & Twycross, R. (Eds.) (1994). *An introduction to palliative care.* Oxford: Sorbell.

Gumley, V. (1992). The development of hospice/palliative care in Russia: A nurse education programme. *European Journal of Cancer Care, 1,* 4.

Gumley, V. (1994). *Russia's expanding hospice network.* London: St. Christopher's Hospice Information Service.

Karajaeva, E. (1994). *"Out of Russia."* London: St. Christopher's Hospice Information Service.

Karajaeva, E. (1995). Hospice development in Tula Oblast. *Medicinskaya Gazette, 65,* 8.

Nokov, G. (1995). Talk given at Chelmsford Hospice, United Kingdom.

St. Gregory's (1993). *The Moscow sisterhood.* [Video.]

Telyukov, A. V. (1990). *Soviet health data.* Moscow: Institute for Economic Studies.

World Health Organization. (1990). *World health statistics.* Geneva: Author.

World Health Organization. (1993). *Cancer pain relief and palliative care.* Geneva: Author.

Zorza, R., & Zorza, V. (1981). *A way to die: Living to the end.* Sphere Books Ltd.

# 17

# Hospice in Spain

Joan Hunt and Marisa Martin, M. D.

## THE BEGINNINGS OF HOSPICE IN SPAIN'S
## COSTA DEL SOL

The name CU DE CA is derived from the legal title, "Asociacion para CUiados DEI CAncer" (Association for Cancer Care). The motto of the organization is "a special kind of caring." Its goal is to build Spain's first independent hospice, and meanwhile to provide home care to terminally ill cancer patients in need. CUDECA's symbol represents the figure of a person whose arms and heart are reaching out to give loving care. At present CUDECA is giving professional palliative home care and counseling to a growing number of patients and their relatives. Thanks to the generous financial support of the international population of the Costa del Sol, funds are being banked toward the estimated total of 200–250 million pesetas (between $1.6 and $2 million in U.S. dollars) needed to open a 15-bed hospice on land which, hopefully, will be donated privately or by a local council.

The hospice project started early in 1991. Fred Hunt, a retired Briton, died of terminal cancer in the Red Cross (Cruz Roja) Hospital in Malaga, Spain's fifth largest city (population 700,000) and the capital of Malaga province in which the Costa del Sol mainly lies. The hospital had a small palliative unit of 12 beds which had been opened in October, 1990. It was the first hospital in Andalucia to have a unit of this type. The alternatives were to pay for private treatment, which is too expensive for many people, or, for the non-Spanish, to return to their homelands.

Two of the Spanish doctors with whom Joan Hunt, wife of the deceased patient, became very friendly were Dra. Marisa Martin Rosello and Dra. Susana Pascual

Laveria. Both had visited hospices in England and had been very impressed by what they saw and learned about palliative care. They agreed it would be wonderful if there was a hospice in Spain similar to those in in the United Kingdom.

Following the death of her husband, Joan Hunt received large donations of money from family and friends in his memory. She donated this money to the Red Cross Hospital as a token of her appreciation for the excellent medical care given. Two British ladies heard about this donation and decided they would also like to help. Flora Willis and Iris Dober had for a number of years held an annual luncheon to raise funds for charity. They contacted Joan and told her that their next charity luncheon would be for her fund. However, by that time Joan had come to realize the limitations of developing the Palliative Unit of the Red Cross Hospital into something along the lines of hospices existing in the U.K. She therefore took the opportunity to invite her doctor friends and others who were sympathetic to the cause, and 25 assorted residents of the Costa del Sol community met at the buffet luncheon on September 8, 1991. Among them were doctors and nurses from the Red Cross Palliative Care Unit. Also present, among others, was a British physician, Anthony Crichton-Smith, who had cared for Fred Hunt, and Susan Hannam, a UK qualified nurse with Spanish convalidation who three years later would become the Medical team Coordinator for CUDECA.

Joan Hunt explained to her guests her desire to have a hospice based on UK and international standards, and her willingness to devote her time to fulfill this ambition if those present would support her. Their response was unanimous, and all signed a sheet of paper pledging their support to help raise money to build the hospice. The first donation of 50,000 pesetas toward the project was raised at that luncheon from a raffle and the sale of homemade jams and other articles. Joan Hunt remembers driving back home to nearby Fuengirola and suddenly being overwhelmed by the enormity of the task she had undertaken and her public commitment to achieving success. So shaken was she that she pulled into a lay-by to stop, think, and recover. For the first of many occasions to come, she felt strengthened and encouraged by the thought that she was doing the right thing and that "someone" was going to support and guide her.

The first task was to have the charity registered as a legal institution. Hunt was fortunate in having a Spanish lawyer, Ricardo Urdiales Galvez, as a close neighbor and friend. He immediately agreed to help after hearing her explanation of the hospice concept. The original luncheon group met with the lawyer on numerous occasions to agree on the wording of the statutes. They were all signatories to the document as founding members of the association. Legal registration was received in July, 1992, which was the shortest period of time ever for statutes to be approved and a charity registered in Spain.

A Board of Management was elected in accordance with the statutes at the first formal meting of the newly registered association, at which Joan Hunt was elected president. Elected to work with her were four Spanish members—the vice president, lawyer, treasurer, and medical director—together with the secretary from Holland, vice secretary from America, the spiritual adviser and fund-raising director—both British—and an American heading up the Hospice Project. All the founding members remain very much involved with the various activities of CUDECA. Four are on the Board of Management, which makes a truly international body of people working together to fulfill the pledge to open a hospice in the Province of Malaga.

An "awareness campaign" started with a press release about the local theater benefit production of *Gypsy*. After the financial success of the show, there followed other fundraising events that resulted in large donations, a deluge of support from volunteers, and requests for help from victims of cancer and their relatives.

## CUDECA IN OPERATION

Priority was given to organizing a palliative home care team consisting of two doctors and two nurses, plus volunteers as yet untrained and therefore only available to help with basic tasks. At that time, the doctors and nurses gave their time without claiming any expenses, and as the funds mounted it was time to get the charity properly organized.

The demands on the limited medical services rapidly increased, as did the fundraising efforts. It became increasingly obvious to Joan Hunt that she could no longer run the organization from her own home, as she had done for the first 18 months. Dr. Marisa Martin and Joan Hunt spent many months looking at property, and eventually settled on a house which suited their needs. Negotiations ran smoothly; however, on the day before the deposit was to be paid a higher offer was made and accepted by the seller. Both ladies were bitterly disappointed, but Ricardo Urdiales Galves, CUDECA's lawyer, assured them that something else would turn up and it did. Shortly after, he located a nearby office suite that would be on the market at a low price. CUDECA purchased the suite and opened the center in October, 1993.

Today, Centro CUDECA consists of a large entrance/reception hall, which houses a lending library of books relating to cancer and bereavement in several languages; an office and consulting room for the medical personnel; a storage room for medical equipment; kitchen facilities; a main office equipped with a powerful computer, on which all the accounts and records are kept; and a conference room for meetings and volunteer training and lectures. Centro CUDECA is open daily and is entirely staffed by volunteers, who are kept very busy receiving inquiries from patients or families asking for help; coordinating the volunteers; organizing the training courses; maintaining liaisons with the various fundraising activities; and generally controlling all administrative areas of CUDECA, which includes providing translation requirements.

There are three basic ways patients are referred to CUDECA. One is via the Palliative Care Unit of the Red Cross Hospital in Malaga. This PCU has a home care program, which covers only the limits of the city of Malaga because of limited resources. At present, CUDECA's home care team treats patients within the Province of Malaga outside of the city, working closely with the Red Cross Hospital Palliative Care Program. Patients are normally referred to CUDECA at an early stage of treatment, so that palliative care can be of immediate help. This quick response pattern has been achieved through the hard and efficient work carried out by the Red Cross Palliative Care Program, not only in direct services but also in spreading the basic principles of palliative medicine among the health professionals of Malaga.

Another referral route is through other local health professionals, such as doctors and social workers in the public health sector, as well as from private doctors and clinics. CUDECA has made official presentations in local health centers and private clinics to offer our help in the clinical, psychological, and social aspects of caring for terminally ill cancer patients. This service is offered as an extra resource, to help the other care providers but not to take over their work. Generally, this approach is understood and well accepted by other professionals, and the number of patients referred to us is slowly growing. Unfortunately, private doctors still tend to refer patients at a late stage of their illness.

The third main referral point is directly from relatives of the patient or the patients themselves. As time goes by, more people have become aware of our project. It is now not unusual for people to come to the center asking for help for themselves, a close relative, or a friend in any stage of the illness, even from the moment of the diagnosis. Counselling facilities are also available and developing because of this need. We are also aware of the need for palliative care for people with AIDS, and this is a dimension of our service that will be receiving increasing attention.

Ever since the first press release, there has been a steady flow of volunteers of all nationalities. Now there are 20–30 annually who are interviewed by a former personnel manger of a major UK company, who makes an assessment of their skills and character. Those selected for direct patient care attend the monthly training courses, which are conducted by professionals—doctors, psychologists, and nurses. The introduction session is repeated during the year to enable new volunteers to slot into the scheduled courses. Other volunteers who may not be selected for direct patient care are recommended to help in the charity shops or in the center, or with fundraising activities and the like. New patient contact comes either by word mouth, from local health centers, or through the Red Cross Hospital in Malaga, whose work is basically limited to the City of Malaga because, as was noted above, they do not have the finances or personnel to carry out home visits outside of the City.

The medical coordinator visits the patient and family either alone or with a doctor on the same day as the initial request for help is received, or, certainly, within 24 hours. She makes an initial assessment of the needs and sets up the necessary program for the doctors, nurses, and volunteers that will be required. There are support groups for both the volunteers and the medical teams, so that all are fully informed and counseled about the situation regarding patients, techniques applied, and developments.

The international nature of CUDECA's work is reflected by the nationalities of the many patients treated: British (47%), Spanish (48%), German, French, Belgian, Swedish, Dutch, Portugese, American, and Danish (combined 15%). CUDECA has cared for them through their hard-working and dedicated palliative medical team of three doctors, four nurses, and a psychologist. This team is strengthened by volunteers, some of whom have received diplomas for attending the required number of monthly training sessions.

A bereavement counseling support group meets fortnightly for the families of deceased patients. Three months after the death of a patient, the beraved relatives are invited to join this support group.

## HOSPICE CARE IN AN INTERNATIONAL RESORT AREA

To understand the context within which CUDECA functions, it is necessary to know something about the unique international population of the Costa del Sol and appreciate something about traditional Spanish values. With possibly the best climate in Europe, it has attracted many Europeans and Americans.

The first to see the potential was Prince Alfonso Hohenlohe of Liechtenstein, who invited his wealthy German friends to join in starting to develop Marbella in the 1950's. Then came the British and an influx of other nationalities, particularly those escaping from the cold winters of Scandinavia. Many holidaymakers of all European nationalities, having enjoyed the climate, the Spanish hospitality, and the facilities for all kinds of sports, return regularly or retire or buy a property for winter living in what has been described as "the California of Europe."

Andalucia has seen many invasions. It was occupied by the Moors for around 500 years—but during the last 40 years, the biggest invasion yet has occurred, for it is estimated that around 250,000 non-Spanish live there for all or much of the year. There are 3 million arrivals a year at Malaga airport and the total foreign and Spanish population of the Costa del Sol is around 1 million.

All this has created opportunities for both the Spanish and the non-Spanish to set up businesses to provide the international community and visitors with the goods and services they require. In consequence, there are young, income-earning foreigners, whose children are growing up bilingual, as well as those in their "golden years" and some not so old, as retirement ages drop, including a few who have made their fortunes early in life. Apart from those working people, many of these foreigners of whatever nationality have something in common—time on their hands to help a good cause. In addition, this international population has created its own media—English, German, Dutch, and Scandinavian magazines, two free weekly English newspapers, three local radio stations, and two local TV stations catering for the Spanish- and English-speaking communities.

This profusion of clubs and media means that there are excellent channels of communication along the Costa del Sol from which CUDECA is benefiting enormously in harnessing the goodwill of many foreigners, thanks to the support it is receiving from the clubs in raising funds and the media in publicizing its activities.

However, there has also been another strong influencing factor. Traditionally, the predominantly Roman Catholic Spanish have a strong belief in the importance of the family unit. One has only to see them at a drawn-out Sunday lunch or picnic to appreciate this devotion to family life . . . mother, father, children, grandparents, uncles, aunts, and their offspring, all relishing the food and enjoying the company of a close-knit family outing.

Family ties have been challenged recently by migration from rural areas to seek work in the towns or a greater mobility of labor. But when it comes to looking after the sick and elderly, the family will rally around. Many would regard allowing an elderly relative to enter a residential home as a social stigma. In addition, there is no Spanish translation of the word "hospice." This nearest is *hospicio*—an orphanage. The words used for hospice are *residencia geriatrica* or *de ancianos*, with the connotation that they are for the old and the poor.

Furthermore, there is no Spanish translation of the word "cancer." The same international word is used, and many Spanish people still fear to utter the word and often do not want to recognize its existence. There is also the interesting contribution of the happy, friendly Andalucian character. Many believe in telling people only what they think they want to hear. Giving bad news is a task that is strenuously avoided. For instance, the plumber may say he will come "mañana" because that is what you want to hear. He will not give you the bad news that you may be lucky to see him next week!

Traditionally, dying people in Spain stayed at home, surrounded by their family, including children. As a result of this practice, the children had early knowledge of death. Dying people would be suppported by friends and neighbors and treated by the family doctor. The patients were the first to know or to feel that they were going to die. This knowledge led to a deeply emotional period of forgiving and saying goodbye. Dying people would also ask their families to carry out their last wishes. Spain being a predominantly Catholic country, it was customary for the local priest to be called to give the last rites and blessing. He would have walked to the home, preceded by an altar boy ringing the bells so that the neighbors would know that the end was near. The process of dying was considered as a natural part of human existence.

Over the last two or three decades, however, these old traditions have been changing. Now the family tries to hide the reality from the patient and from each other. The children are no longer present in the household, and consequently are not so deeply aware of how death occurs. With its self-protective attitude, the family does not ask the priest to come to the house until the patient is very close to death, because they fear his presence would frighten the patient and he would realize he was dying.

Nowadays, the majority of people do not die at home—the ideal place to hide the dying is the hospital. Dying people are taken into hospital on their own initiative or the family's, in either case seeking modern technology and curative treatment.

And so terminal patients are not always been told the bad news of cancer. They may be told instead that they have bronchitis, a chest complaint, a bad throat, a stomach disorder, or any other less disturbing story. In fact, a lot of the Associations time was spent discussing the use of the word cancer in its title. This fear to speak openly of cancer and death is changing, but the concept of a hospice and admission of the reality of cancer is still shunned by many. Communication is relatively easy with the large number of foreigners who know what a hospice is and can speak of cancer. It is from this quarter that much of the startup funds were received.

It is hoped that the Spanish business community will become more involved in providing donations and to this end, early in 1995, the first *Boletin de CUDECA*, a four-page newspaper, was printed in both languages. However, the backbone of CUDECA's fundraising presently comes from their four second-hand charity shops, the first being close to the Centro CUDECA in Fuengirola, the premises being originally loaned, rent-free, for a year by a Spanish doctor. Two others opened in 1994 along the coast in Torremolinos and Torre del Mar, and the fourth opened in 1995 in the inland village of Coin. Significantly, the Spanish attitude towards the work of CUDECA was demonstrated by the mayor of Coin's opening the shop himself, and inviting the British couple who run it to help teach English at the town's Institute. The shops raise 30% of CUDECA's revenue, enabling every peseta from donations and fundraising events to be placed in the hospice fund, earning a good rate of interest. Their continuous growth and successes provide all the revenue to meet the cost of running the office, training volunteers, financing the palliative home care service, investing in more fundraising projects, and contributing a surplus to the hospice fund.

Significantly the shops, in which 70–80 volunteers work, receive significant public support, both through donations of articles for sale and through purchase. The growth of CUDECA's support is reflected by the fact that in 1994 the gross income was 27.4 million pesetas, compared to 20.5 million pesetas to the end of 1993. Donations, fundraising events, the "In memory" fund, plus collecting tins and bricks amounted to 14 million pesetas, of which 5 million came from the sale of a property donated by the widower of a patient.

The growing status of CUDECA is reflected by the ever-increasing number of national and international organizations with which it is linked. CUDECA is a member of SECPAL—Sociedad Espanola de Cuidados Paliativos—which, in turn, is affiliated with the European Association of Cancer Care. The medical team presented a paper on its home care service and plans to open an inpatient hospice at the first International SECPAL Congress to be held in Barcelona in December, 1995. The Junta de Andalucia has recognized CUDECA as being a charity-providing health care service. In the UK, CUDECA is a member of the prestigious St. Christopher's Overseas Hospice Information Service, from whom they have received a great deal of help and advice. They have also developed a very friendly relationship with many hospices in the UK, either from meeting representatives at congresses; through encounturs with residents and visitors to the coast whose families are involved with hospices in their own country, and also via CUDECA staff visiting hospices close to their home towns when they make return trips to visit their families or friends.

# THE PERSONAL SIDE OF THE STORY:
# TWO CASE HISTORIES

Each patient's experience is unique and has its own story. Here are two examples.

## DRM

DRM was a 75-year-old Spanish man, married and with 7 children, who was diagnosed as having lung cancer. He lived with his wife who was his principal caregiver, a widowed daughter whose husband had died of cancer, and her 15-year-old son. DRM had worked in a bank until retirement age. Two of his daughters who lived as far away as Madrid came regularly to help and support their mother.

For many years, DRM had been a diabetic and a heavy smoker. The diabetes was controlled by diet and oral medication. The smoking had produced chronic obstructive respiratory disease. He experienced two cerebrovascular accidents 9 months apart, leaving him with hemiparesis in his upper left limb. Six months after the second CVA, he presented with chest pain, fever, loss of weight and appetite, and weakness. DRM was admitted to a private clinic with a provisional diagnosis of pneumonia. Further investigation led to the diagnosis of small cell carcinoma of upper left bronchus with mediastinal bilateral adenopatia. At that time there was no evidence of metastasis.

Following consultation with the oncologist, it was decided that curative treatment was not possible because of his age and previous illnesses. DRM was referred to the PCU of the Red Cross Hospital in Malaga. The family attended the first outpatient appointment and were informed about his situation. It was then agreed to refer DRM to CUDECA for home care, as at that time he was living outside the city of Malaga.

During the first visit of the CUDECA home care team, they found the family to be very anxious and insistent that the patient continue to think that he had only a respiratory tract infection. His wife and children reaffirmed the suggestion that he should not be told the true diagnosis, as this would only produce more suffering with which he would not be able to cope. The family was obviously very sad about the imminent death of the father figure, as they had had several previous experiences of a death by cancer. In addition to the daughter's husband, the wife of one DRM's sons had died of cancer, leaving a young family. This death had been difficult, with little symptom control. The family assumed that DRM would also suffer a painful death. In spite of their anxieties, the family wanted to look after the patient, and they each made a committment to support their mother and help with the care of the father. Therefore, no CUDECA volunteers were required to support the home situation.

The patient was able to get up and move around the house with the help of a stick. He was weak, anorexic, and constipated, and needed assistance with washing and dressing, complaining of headaches and excessive sweating and pain in the chest. Treatment was started and adjusted through successive visits, using analgesics, bronchodilators, cortisone, stool softeners, and enemas. DRM received many visits from the CUDECA home care team, some for symptom control but many just to support the family, who often needed more help than he did. He then moved back into Malaga City with his wife and widowed daughter, where his condition slowly deteriorated.

DRM indicated both to his family and the home care team that he was aware of his terminal condition. His symptome were well-controlled at home, but he felt he was dying. Four days before his death, he was admitted to hospital on the request of his wife, because she felt she would not be able to cope with the final stage. She gathered together all her sons and her daughter and had them by DRM's side in his last days. He died peacefully, surrounded by all his family.

The final visits from the CUDECA home care team were to his wake and to the funeral. DRM's widow and daughter have since become members of CUDECA. All his clothes were donated to the benefit shop, and a substantial donation was made to the CUDECA hospice fund.

# NH

One of our first patients was NH, a 78-year-old British lady with a diagnosis of breast cancer. Her cancer had been diagnosed 11 years previously, when a lumpectomy had been performed, followed by chemotherapy and radiotherapy. Eight years later she developed pulmonary metastasis. At the time of her first contact with CUDECA, NH's medical condition also included chronic anemia, chronic arthritis, deafness, and hypothyroidism related to previous treatment. Her 80-year-old husband was her only caregiver. He had previously had a CVA with residual left hemiparesia. It was NH's second marriage; she had a son from her first marriage who lived in Canada and had no contact with his mother.

The couple had been resident in Spain for three years and lived in their own apartment with very difficult access and no telephone. It was on the third floor, with no lift, and isolated in the country. Although they had a car, it was difficult for the husband to drive. They were pensioners who had owned a market garden in England. They had no friends or relatives in Spain and neither spoke Spanish. Consequently, they were unaware of the bureaucratic process required to transfer their British health system entitlement to Spain.

The first contact with CUDECA was made directly by NH's husband. It was very apparent that the social problems were much more important at that time than her physical condition, which was quite stable. With the help of CUDECA volunteers, the couple moved to a rented apartment on the seafront, with shops and restaurants nearby, in an area where it was easy to walk and meet people. (The proceeds from the sale of their original apartment were donated to CUDECA by the express wish of both the patient and the husband.) Another objective of the move was to make it easier for the volunteers to have daily contact to ensure that regular assistance was given for both the social and health problems of the couple.

Four CUDECA volunteers helped them during the illness. They helped with the cooking and ironing, went to the local doctor for prescriptions, and would take the husband to the doctor when he needed medical checkups. They would also take NH and her husband on shopping trips and out for coffee, or just for sight-seeing rides. In a word, the volunteers became friends.

During the two-year period of her illness, NH had to be admitted twice to the PCU of the Red Cross Hospital in Malaga. The first time was for symptom control, breathlessness, and a respiratory infection, which improved with intensive treatment. After one week, she was able to return home to continue under the care of the CUDECA medical team and volunteers. NH was able to celebrate her 80th birthday at home with her husband and volunteers.

On the occasion of her second admission to the hospital, she had become confused and had generally deteriorated because of the tumor growth in the lung. NH was very worried about how her husband was going to manage and she asked the volunteers if they would continue to look after him. When they assured her that they would do so, she relaxed and died peacefully three days later. The volunteers helped the husband through the bereavement period and still continue to assist him, more than a year and a half after the death of his wife.

After the death of NH, her husband did not want to have a funeral service. He arranged for her body to be cremated without a ceremony. The team who had been involved in her care felt a sense of loss with the need to say goodbye. With the husband's knowledge, they got together in the gardens of a local church, which has magnificent views of the Mediterranean and the mountains, because they knew it was a place she loved to visit. They selected and read aloud "The Soldier" by Rupert Brooke (1914/1985), which had been one of her favorite poems. This is the well-known poem that begins:

> If I should die, think only this of me:
>> That there's some corner of a foreign field
> That is for ever England. . . .

And concludes:

> Her sights and sounds; dreams happy as her day;
>> And laughter, learnt of friends, and gentleness,
> In hearts at peace, under an English heaven.

## FACING NEW CHALLENGES

As CUDECA's work becomes even better known, the demands on its professional medical services continue to increase. In 1995 the first full-time member of staff—Susan Hannam—was appointed as medical team coordinator. Part-time work was no longer sufficient to meet the requests for service that CUDECA strives to provide:

- More bereavement counseling,
- More modern techiques to absorb through training courses,
- More money to reach the hospice fund target as soon as possible, and
- More evaluation and the gathering of ongoing knowledge from research into pain control and symptom relief.

Thankfully, the helping hands are ever increasing to enable CUDECA to continue to provide a special kind of caring.

## REFERENCE

Brooke, R. (1985: origin, 1914). The soldier. In J. Sicken (Ed.), *World War I Poetry*. 2nd edition. Harmound, Millberg England: Penguin Books Limited.

# Asia

# 18

# Hospice Development in China: "Like Green Bamboo Shoots in the Spring"

Anthony Smith, MD, and Douglas Zuefu Zhu, MD

## THE START OF HOSPICE WORK IN CHINA—THE PROMISE OF SPRING

"Providing quality care for terminally ill patients not only safeguards human dignity, but also lightens the burden of their families and working units." This sentiment was presented at the East-West International Conference on Hospice Care, held in Tianjin in 1992 by Minzhang Chen, Minister of Public Health of China and a highly respected professor of medicine. Chen further stated that "Hospice care is a component of developing social productive forces, and a kind of philanthropic act with hundreds of advantages but no single harm. Therefore, the Ministry will work out the necessary regulations to facilitate the healthy development of the cause of hospice care in China" (Chen, 1993, p. 63).

The hospice movement in China started in the summer of 1988 with the establishment of the Hospice Research Center at Tianjin Medical College [currently Tianjin Medical University] by Yitai Tsuei, M.D., Vice President of the college, and Michael T. C. Hwang, Ed.D., former Vice President of Oklahoma City University. This project was initiated 2 months after the first invited lecture on hospice care given by George S. Lair, Ph.D., an American hospice psychologist and president of the East-West Death Education Association (Zhu, 1993).

There is no equivalent term in Chinese for the English word "hospice." "Hospice care" is translated as "linzhong guanhuai" (terminal care) in the mainland, "anning zhaogu" (peaceful care) in Taiwan, and "shanzhong fuwu" (well-ending service) in Hong Kong. Each of these translations not only has the same basic meaning as the original term in English, but also indicates the moral value of caring for dying persons in traditional Chinese culture.

The concept of hospice care, therefore, is not a totally imported value from the Western World, but an integration of the traditional Chinese culture and the philosophy of the modern hospice movement initiated by Dame Cicely Saunders in 1967. A wealth of thought on caring for dying persons in terms of ancient philosophy, social customs, morals, and medical practice can be found in Chinese literature dating thousand of years in the past. The hospice movement in China is developing within this distinctively Chinese background. This perspective is noted also by Qi-ao Qian, physicist and Mayor of Tianjin, and Shouli Shi, a Chinese Air Force physician.

> China is a great nation that has a thousand-year history of civilization and splendid national culture. Although hospice care in this country is a new branch of science and a new concept for most Chinese people, the soruce of the spirit of revolutionary humanitarianism and the glorious moral faith of human being embodied by the modern hospice movement can also be traced back to the traditional Chinese culture (Qian, 1992, p. 2).

Our current practice indicates that the development of hospice in China has a deep social, economic, cultural, historical, and political basis (Shi & Li, 1992, p. 438).

Although many terminal patients make every effort to find a miraculous care, many others "turn home." This decision involves withdrawing from aggressive treatments in favor of alternative, nonaggressive medical approaches and/or comfort care provided by the primary caregivers. "Turning home" is a particularly common decision in the vast rural areas of China. Unfortunately, however, most dying patients suffer physical, psychological, and spiritual pain during their last journey of life because quality care is not available to them.

One of the major problems before the hospice movement started in China was that health care professionals did not realize it was their responsibility to provide palliative or comfort care for dying persons and their families. Instead, the professionals believed that they could do nothing but attempt to cure the patient. As recently as 1985, a visitor to China observed that "Palliative care as we know it is unknown in China. Aggressive treatment is kept up right to the moment of death. . . . If by chance a patient discovers that he or she is terminal, every effort is made to encourage the patient to keep on fighting" (Morgan, 1986, pp. 267–268).

The change in atmosphere between 1985 and 1988 is striking. This change had its roots in the inquiring mind of one man, Dr. Yitai Tsuei—a physiologist, medical educator, and author of ten books including *Hospice Care: Theory and Practice* (1992). His interest in developments in the world of medicine had led him to listen eagerly to reports of the new principles of palliative care which had been reaching China through such people as Dr. Hwang, who had completed a multicultural hospice research project on death education at Drake University in Des Moines, Iowa under the direction of Prof. Lair. Dr. Hwang had published a book on hospice care in Taiwan, where he was in contact with the staff of Mackay Memorial Hospital. In February, 1990, that hospital started the first hospice service in Taiwan under the leadership of its Vice Director, Rev. Dr. David Chung.

These ideas needed to be explored in China as well. Accordingly, Dr. Tsuei founded the Hospice Research Center with the first donations of 50,000 yuan (about $10,000 US) from Dr. Hwang, 1,000 yuan from Ms. Guiying Wang, president of the Tianjin Nursing Association, and 50,000 yuan from Tianjin Medical University. Dr. Tsuei became director. Dr. Hwang was made an honorary director, along with Prof. Xianzhong Wu, M. D., a medical expert well known for his integration of traditional Chinese and Western medicine. Three Vice Directors, including Douglas Zuefu Zhu, M. D., and nine research faculty members were also appointed.

Information was sought wherever it might be available, including the Hospice Information Service at St. Christopher's Hospice in London, which responded to a request for details of hospice development. Dr. Lair and Dr. Hwang were invited to visit China to work at the Center as visiting professors. A series of research projects was conducted between 1989 and 1992. These included a survey of 4,000 Chinese residents, 1348 medical and nursing professionals, and 1053 college and university students. The respondents were asked about their attitudes toward death, dying, and terminal care. This survey contributed to a better understanding of the culture and experience of death, dying, and terminal care in China.

The new concept of hospice care needed to be disseminated throughout China, especially among health care professionals. In 1990 a hospice education and survey project was carried out by the Hospice Research Center. Four faculty members travelled to more than ten provinces and cities to introduce the concept of hospice care to the local health care professionals, and to investigate the status of terminal care in those areas. Based on this project, the first National Conference and Workshop on Hospice Care was held in Tianjin in March, 1991. This meeting succeeded in bringing nationwide attention to hospice care for the first time.

Perhaps coincidentally, the World Health Organization's Cancer and Palliative Care Unit was cooperating with various focal groups in China to develop a national palliative care program. A first national cancer pain relief and palliative care workshop was organized by the WHO in association with the Ministry of Public Health and the Chinese Academy of Medical Sciences in Guangzhou in November, 1990. It was attended by more than a hundred doctors, as well as seven nurses and a single pharmacist. The participants represented many areas of China. Palliative care principles were discussed and the participants planned to fan out through China to spread information on cancer pain relief and palliative care (MacDonald, Sun, & Teoh, 1992).

## "LIKE BAMBOO SHOOTS"—A CHINESE MOVEMENT SPROUTS

Interest spread fast. A nursing home in Shanghai was converted to hospice-type care, and so began the Nan Hui Hospice. A ward was designated for hospice care in a large public lung disease hospital in Tianjin, and in four other hospitals associated with the Tianjin Medical College.

By early 1992 there were six hospice units in China known to the Hospice Research Center. A year later there were another 45. Currently, hospice services are available or are being developed in more than two-thirds of the provinces, autonomous regions, and municipalities of China.

It was Prof. Tsuei who commented that hospices were "sprouting and growing like green bamboo shoots in the spring!"

## WHY SHOULD HOSPICE CARE BE RELEVANT IN CHINA?

Sun, Jian, and Wang (1992) observed that "Special institutions have been set up to deal with birth, development, and illness, but, unreasonably, not with death." To Sun (1993), hospice care for dying patients in China was not only feasible, but necessary, for the following reasons:

1. There is pressure from the increasing population of dying persons. Chinese constitute almost one-fourth of the world's population. The number of elderly people is increasing, and there are now more and more critically ill people who cannot take care of themselves and have no one to look after them.
2. There is pressure from society. China is short of hospitals, hospital beds, and doctors. Therefore, it is difficult for patients to consult a doctor or to be hospital-

ized. Patients in the terminal stage of cancer are not admitted to hospitals, so they often die in emergency wards, at the same time interfering with treatment of other seriously ill patients.

3. There is desire on the part of the people. With the wider dissemination of death education, the people have become better prepared psychologically for death. The fact that Nan Hui Hospice in Shanghai was quickly accepted by the public shows that it is in conformity with the popular desire.

4. It is financially feasible. Although China is not a rich country, hospice care for the dying does not require a great deal of expensive equipment or special experts, and is therefore financially feasible. Hospice care charges only a relatively small amount of money, which is within the means of the patients and their units.

For all these reasons, it was argued, hospice care for the dying should be included in the urban medical network (Sun & Wang, 1992).

# RESEARCHING HOSPICE PRACTICE—EXPLORING THE GROWTH

The first East-West International Conference on Hospice Care was organized by the Hospice Research Center in 1992, in association with the East-West Death Education Association, the Hospice of Central Iowa, and the Society for the Promotion of Hospice Care in Hong Kong. Held in Tianjin, the conference attracted 400 senior doctors, nurses, and medical administrators from 29 of the 30 provinces, autonomous regions, and municipalities of China. Several senior members of the Army, Navy, and Air Force Medical Services were also included.

In preparation for the conference, 1364 professional papers related to palliative, terminal, and hospice care were submitted from many parts of China. Four hundred and eighty papers were published in Chinese and the abstracts of 74 of these were translated into English for publication. Some of these are quoted in this chapter. In addition, Dr. Tsuei and Dr. Hwang coauthored a book on hospice care in Chinese, and synopses of the papers from the invited speakers were also published.

A year later, the Research Center organized a second national conference, this time in Yantai, Shandong Province. The National Hospice Society of China was established and Dr. Tsuei was elected as the first president. Again, significant papers were presented and the growth of the Chinese hospice movement was further documented.

Sixteen seminars and workshops in six different provinces and cities were organized by the Research Center in the early 1990s. Two were arranged after each of the conferences mentioned above, and led by Dr. Anthony Smith, Director of Studies at St. Christopher's Hospice, London. Eight other conferences were led by Prof. Lair. The experiences of both Eastern and Western caregivers were shared at these conferences. Approximately 2,000 senior doctors, nurses, and health care administrators were trained in the principles and skills of hospice care. Visits were also arranged whenever possible to enable participants to see some of the hospice units. A survey of the effects of the hospice seminars held in Tianjin in 1991 and 1992 found that significant positive attitudinal changes had occurred among the medical and nursing professionals (Lair & Zhu, 1993).

In 1993 a new required course on hospice care was included for the medical students in the general practitioner major at Tianjin Medical College, and for nursing students at Tianjin Health Care Professionals College. A textbook for the course (Zhu, 1993) was also published.

## HOSPICE MODELS IN CHINA

Currently there are four basic hospice models existing in China.

### 1. Hospital-based Hospice Wards or Units

According to 1992 statistics, China has 2,744,000 beds distributed among more than 15,000 hospitals at the county level and above, and in more than 40,000 health centers at the township level. These facilities serve 1,170 million Chinese people in the mainland (Sun, 1993). Although the average number of beds per thousand population in China was only 0.426, the rate of empty beds in many hospitals has continued to rise in recent years. This increase in vacancy rate is thought to be attributable either to increasing success of the disease prevention movement, or to the shortage of medical resources.

It was possible, then, for some hospitals to transform some regular beds into hospice beds. The health care reform policy in China also encourages hospitals to develop new programs to serve the community based on its current needs. This policy has facilitated the development of hospital-based hospice wards or units.

The major advantage of developing a hospital-based hospice war or unit has been the efficiency in time and resource management. Most hospice programs in China have been developed on this model.

### 2. Nursing Home-based Hospice Services

There is a great need in China today to provide all forms of nursing care, including hospice care. Nan Hui Hospice in Shanghai was developed on this model. This facility is still known to the pubic as Nan Hui Nursing Home. In Beijing, the hospice unit of Chao Yang Men Hospital was developed in a similar way. Additionally, some nursing homes have simply incorporated the principles of hospice care into their patient services, instead of establishing a separate hospice ward or unit.

## 3. Independent Hospices

Currently there are three types of independent hospice in China:

(a) A for-profit business eatablished by existing healthcare institutes or other nonprofit organizations. These for-profit businesses must be separated from the nonprofit units.

(b) A for-profit business founded by other profit enterprises, individuals, or as a joint venture.

(c) Nonprofit public health services. A project to establish a public hospice was approved by the Public Health Bureau of Gulou District, Nanjing in 1993.

## 4. Home-based Hospice Services

Home-based hospice services have been developed in several provinces and municipalities, such as Tianjin and Sichuan. They are not very popular. It is believed that many home-based hospice services are categorized as regular home health care services, instead of being presented as a new hospice care program. Inconvenient living conditions, such as crowding and lack of home telephones and private automobiles, are barriers to developing 24-hour inservice home-based hospice programs.

## CURRENT PERSPECTIVES ON THE CHINESE MODEL OF HOSPICE CARE

Zhou and Mi (1992) of Kunming General Hospital have observed that hospice care presents a new challenge for nurses who need to seek "a Chinese model which is applicable to the Chinese people. . . . Hospice care should proceed in actual Chinese conditions, and in accord with the national custom and the present situation of nursing. We cannot imitate indiscriminately the foreign model and methods."

Nevertheless, the main characteristics of a developing model are recognizable (Xu & Xu, 1992). Hospices should:

1. Serve all the people.
2. Provide reasonable and inexpensive services.
3. Provide both central services (free-standing hospices) and dispersion (in-home) care.
4. Allow religion to play a part in the service, in keeping with the preferences of the dying people; and their relatives. (pp. 402–403)

Zhao (1992) suggests that hospice care wards in general hospitals, establish specific hospice care facilities; use existing clinics, both rural and urban; and encourage the development of private hospice care clinics.

Despite the barriers to hospice care at home in China, some favorable observations have been made. After three years of home hospice care experience, Wang (1992) observed that

> This kind of hospice care model has been well received by both the dying patients and their relatives. . . . Our finds are that hospice care given at home is in accordance with the situation in China. [it] prolongs patients' life expectancies, makes everything convenient both for the patients and their family members and . . . lightens the financial burden for the persons concerned and society.

What is being aimed for? Wu (1992) states that

> We always adopt palliative treatment, control the patients' pain, offer them better service, regulate their diets, and increase their nutrition. Hospice care also includes working for the patients' relatives, persuading them to restrain their grief and letting them become part of the hospice care team. Immediately before their death, we have to try our best to help the patients feel happy. Their suffering should be alleviated physiologically, spiritually, and psychologically, and their dignity protected.

Chinese medicine at present makes use of three strands: traditional Chinese medicine, Qigong practice (a form of medication and body-mind exercise), and Western allopathic medicine. Hospice care readily makes use of all three forms of practice, and has therefore proved highly acceptable in China. Dr. Li Wei, director of the Song Tang Hospital (the first hospice in Beijing) told one of the authors that using all three methods allowed the care to be "reliable—like a stool with three legs!"

## THE BAMBOO SHOOTS THEMSELVES

Come, visit a Chinese hospice!

Second Affiliated Hospital of Tianjin Medical College is a large facility with 836 beds. Above the door of its hospice ward is a large sign whose Chinese characters apparently mean "Clinical Ward." (The hospice ward in the Tianjin Lung Disease Hospital uses the term "Caring Ward.")

When this ward opened in October, 1990, it had 16 beds. As a result of popular demand, the ward has been enlarged twice, and consists now of 30 beds. Patients reside in rooms with from one to four beds. The staff consists of six doctors, nine nurses, and 15 nurse aides. These caregivers work three shifts a day to cover the ward 24 hours, 7 days a week. In the first 18 months of operation, the staff cared for 190 patients.

The length of stay ranges from 1 day to 6 months, with an average stay of 12 days. Ninety percent of the patients here are cancer sufferers. The most common cancers have been those of liver, lung, stomach, and the esophagus, in that order.

Although patients prefer to die at home if possible, 97 (51%) have died on the ward.

The hospice ward is intended "to reduce pain, to ease comfort, to provide dignity, and to research quality of life." To that end, the hospice ward is more "homelike." The walls are painted in two colors, as distinguished from the monochromatic treatment in the rest of the hospital. This is intended to encourage a different atmosphere. There are also television sets, a radio, and a tape player—unusual provisions for a hospital ward in China. Additionally, the family is allowed to stay with the patient.

We meet a number of patients. Some are obviously very well; some almost unconscious. Most are middle-aged or elderly, but there is one young person whose severe pain problem is being treated. The atmosphere in the ward is peaceful, but active. Overall, pain control seems to be effective. One observes acupuncture needles in place in some patients. Several have intravenous drips, as esophageal and stomach cancer increase the need for nutrition and hydration. We also meet a number of family members for whom the staff is attempting to provide support. In turn, the staff also needs mutual support, as the director observes.

A similar picture prevails in other Chinese hospice units, but the patients are not always cancer sufferers. A significant proportion of patients in other units have had a stroke, or suffer from terminal heart disease or advanced lung diseases. Tuberculosis is among the lung diseases that is found among patients in the hospice ward of the Lung Disease Hospital. Length of stay in such cases tends to be longer. This willingness to provide palliative care for an extended period of time seems to be a reflection of the great concern in China for the support of the elderly infirm.

## AND IN TAIWAN. . . .

At the same time that hospice services were developing in mainland China, similar services were being established in Taiwan at the Mackay Memorial Hospital through the leadership of Rev. David Chung. Physicians, nurses, social workers, and clergy became involved in this holistic care program for terminal cancer patients.

Lai (1994) has reviewed the first 497 patients to be served at this facility. Pain was the most common symptom, and total pain relief was achieved for 80% of the patients. Awareness of dying was evident in 412 (86%). Most of the patients were said to have become aware of the prospect of death through their own observations, but 132 were informed by medical staff.

The hospice team encountered five major problems in its first years of operation: (1) need for more education and training; (2) psychological pressure; (3) management of loss and grief; (4) need for more emotional support for the caregivers; and (5) troubles caused by families' lying to patients.

## ISSUES FOR CHINESE HOSPICE CARE

The future of hospice care in China will depend to some extent on the resolution of issues such as the following:

### 1. Reimbursement for Hospice Care

There is no doubt that hospice care is much needed in China. Given that one-fifth of the world's population lives in China, about 1 million new cases of cancer occur each year. Many of the patients already have cancer at an advanced stage when it is first diagnosed. Unfortunately, there are millions of people in both rural and urban areas who do not have sufficient medical benefits or insurance to cover hospice care: they cannot afford the services they so urgently need. Many Chinese scholars believe that the number one priority for Chinese hospice care should be how to make this service available for all the people who need them.

### 2. Pain Control

The World Health Organization recommends a three-step analgesic ladder. It was found that about half the participants in a hospice conference in Guanzhou were familiar with this recommendation, but "they were substantially fearful of the addictive potential of morphine" (MacDonald et al., 1992, p. 7). Other surveys have confirmed that many Chinese physicians are familiar with the WHO recommendations, but that some hesitate to use morphine when it would be the most effective medication. The strongest analgesic in common use is pethidine (Dolantin), taken orally or sometimes by injection. Some physicians prefer meperidine by injection when the need for pain relief is at its peak (Kerr, 1993). However, some hospice units are beginning to use oral morphine in an effective manner.

Qin (1992) advocates the use of dihydroetorphine (DHE). He describes DHE as "a new narcotic analgesic successfully manufactured in our country which has been approved to be produced by our Government. . . . It is a high potency medicine, and (has) no cross tolerance with morphine. The analgesia of DHE is stronger while the addiction is less." The drawback is that DHE has a short duration of action (only two hours) and has to be given sublingually or by injection. DHE is more acceptable than morphine in China, however—one is still reminded of the opium wars of the previous century. DHE may find a useful place in the opioid armamentarium. But the authors have seen a patient for whom frequent sublingual DHE was not able to control the pain of a spinal tumor, and for whom morphine seemed to be the only hope for relief.

It remains to be seen whether or not morphine will become more acceptable in China and whether or not other effective medications will become available for relieving pain that cannot be managed through other modalities.

## 3. "Telling Patients"

Discussion in hospice seminars has revealed the usual differences between those caring staff—often nurses—who would tell patients their diagnoses and prognoses if the patients showed a desire to know, and those equally caring staff—often doctors—who felt that to tell the patient the diagnosis was to "encourage him or her to give up."

Nevertheless, there was a consensus that the climate of opinion is changing in China with the increasing dissemination of death education. It was also agreed that many more patients are now being informed and supported through their increasing awareness of the terminal nature of their illness.

## 4. Euthanasia

Euthanasia has been the subject of a hot public debate in China since the late 1980s, and has more recently become a major issue. The First Chinese Symposium on Euthanasia was held in Shanghai in 1987. Headline news at that time was a recent case of a young doctor who had provided "euthanasia" for an elderly terminally ill patient at the request of his family. The doctor that had been prosecuted at the instigation of other members of the patient's family. Some health care professionals confused the term linzghonz guanhuai (terminal care) with euthanasia—which itself was translated into Chinese as "happy death." Stimulated both by the controversy and the linguistic confusion, many papers were submitted to the Symposium on the question of whether hospices should approve of euthanasia.

Cases cited during the discussions included the situations of the elderly person who was terminally ill and did not want to be a burden to family or society; the advanced cancer sufferer with a distressing and unrelieved situation; the person in a persistent vegetative state; and the brain-dead person maintained on life support after an accident. It was pointed out that in China the criterion of life was the beating heart, not proof of brain activity. Arguments on the pro and con sides of euthanasia were heard and discussed with care and obvious concern.

Only a year later, however, it had become apparent that Chinese medical ethicists had decided that euthanasia should not be regarded as in any sense a part of palliative care. This opinion made itself known clearly at the Second National Conference on Hospice Care.

## 5. Psychological and Spiritual Care

The psychological care of dying people was a major theme for papers included in the 1992 conference. Zhang's (1992) report from the department of Surgery at Yijishan Hospital not only reflected on the clinical management of 180 dying patients, but also offers a valuable concluding comment on the progress of the concept of holistic hospice care in China.

Zhang emphasized the importance of:

- Observing the patient's condition;
- Coordinating emergency activities when necessary;
- Offering spiritual consolation;
- Respecting the patient's dignity and self-esteem;
- Communicating with patients frequently to alleviate unstable moods; and
- Comforting the family members.

Ther is no doubt that hospice care has made a very effective start in China since 1988, but all agree that there is still much yet to accomplish.

## REFERENCES

Chen, M. (1993). Opening address at the First East-West International Conference on Hospice Care, Tianjin, China (1992). *Proceedings of the Second National Conference on Hospice Care, China* (p. 63). Tianjin: Tianjin Medical University.

Cong, S. (1992). Treatment of progressive carcinous pain with oral medication. *Proceedings of the First East-West International Conference on Hospice Care*. Tianjin: Tianjin Medical University.

Jiao, D., & Liu, J. (1992). Pain control of advanced stage cancer patients. *Proceedings of the First East-West International Conference on Hospice Care*. Tianjin: Tianjin Medical University.

Kerr, D. (1993). Lin zhong guan huai: Terminal care in China. *American Journal of Hospice and Palliative Care*, 18–26.

Lai, Y. (1994). Continuing hospice care of cancer—A three year experience. *Journal of the Formosa Medical Association, 93*, 98–102.

Lair, G. S., & Zhu, D. X. (1993). *Effects of hospice seminars on the attitudes of Chinese health care professionals toward terminal care*. Unpublished manuscript.

MacDonald, N., Yan, S., & Teoh, N. (1992). Initiatives in China. *Palliative Medicine, 6*, 6–8.

Morgan, J. D. (1986). One glimpse of terminal care in China and Japan. *Journal of Palliative Care, 2*, 41–42.

Morgan, J. D. (1986). Death, dying, and bereavement in China and Japan: A brief glimpse. *Death Studies, 10*(3), 265–272.

Mu, W. (1992). A prospect of hospice care. *Proceedings of the First East-West International Conference on Hospice Care*. Tianjin: Tianjin Medical University.

Qian, Q. (1992). Preface. In Y. Tsuei & T. C. Wang (Eds.), *Hospice care: Theory and practice* (pp. 1–2). Beijing: Chinese Medical Science Press.

Qin, B., & Huang, M. (1992). A research progress of high-efficient analgesic dihydroetorphine and its clinical application. *Proceedings of the First East-West International Conference on Hospice Care.* Tianjin: Tianjin Medical University.

Shi, L. (Ed.) (1993). *Medical and health services in China* (p. 438). Beijing: Ministry of Public Health of China.

Shi, S., & Li, S. H. (1992). The hospice model suitable for China and the problems lying ahead of it. *Proceedings of the First East-West International Conference on Hospice Care.* Tianjin: Tianjin Medical University.

Sun, J., & Wang, H. (1992). The necessity and feasibility of hospice care for dying patients in China. *Proceedings of the First East-West International Conference on Hospice Care.* Tianjin: Tianjin Medical University.

Sun, L., Chen, M., Gu, Y., Li. S., & Wang, B. (Eds.) (1993). *Medical and Health Services in China.* Beijing: Ministry of Public Health of China.

Tsuei, Y., & Hwang, M. T. (1992). *Hospice: Theory and Practice.* Beijing: China. Medical-Pharmacentical Science & Technology Publishing House.

Wang, F. (1992). A preliminary study of the family model of hospice care. *Proceedings of the First East-West International Conference on Hospice Care.* Tianjin: Tianjin Medical University.

Wu, W. (1992). A prospect of hospice care. In Secretariat of the First East-West International Conference in Hospice Care (Ed.), *Proceedings of the First East-West International Conference on Hospice Care* (pp. 429–430). Tianjin: Tianjin Medical University.

Xu, Z., & Xu, S. (1992). Developing hospice with China's national condition and folk custom. *Proceedings of the First East-West International Conference on Hospice Care.* Tianjin: Tianjin Medical University.

Zhang, J. (1992). Elementary introduction to the psychological and nursing problems of dying patients. *Proceedings of the First East-West International Conference on Hospice Care.* Tianjin: Tianjin Medical University.

Zhao, F. (1992). A primary review on the mode of hospice care. *Proceedings of the First East-West International Conference on Hospice Care.* Tianjin: Tianjin Medical University.

Zhou, Y., & Mi, J. (1992). Hospice care: A new problem of nursing study. *Proceedings of the First East-West International Conference on Hospice Care.* Tianjin: Tianjin Medical University.

Zhu, X. (1993). *An introduction to hospice care.* Tianjin: Tianjin Medical University.

# 19

# The Hospice Movement in a Chinese Society—A Hong Kong Experience

## Lucy S. T. Chung

Hong Kong is an international city in which the majority of the population is Chinese. A mixture of Chinese and Western ideas influences the people's thinking and their way of life. Attitudes toward death, however, are still very much governed by traditional Chinese beliefs. Many people think that talking about death will bring bad luck. Among Chinese people of the older generation, the attitude towards incurable diseases is distorted by the fear of contagion, as well as the belief that a condition such as cancer is punishment for evildoing in this life or in a previous existence. These beliefs often intensify distress, because patients are faced with possible isolation from family and friends. Furthermore, death rarely takes place at home. Many people have superstitious ideas that a death at home would bring bad luck to the house. For some older people, idol worship and rituals are seen as ways to combat death.

The hospice movement originated, and has been most extensively developed, in the Western world. Palliative care influences attitudes toward dying, the structure of caregiving, and ways of dying. Some hospice concepts are not only unfamiliar, but also differ from the beliefs of many residents of Hong Kong. The experience of hospice development in Hong Kong therefore represents an ideological challenge, as well as an alternative approach to caregiving for terminally ill people and their families.

## INADEQUACY OF CARE

More than 9,000 people die from cancer in Hong Kong each year. Before the hospice approach was introduced, there was no special care for the terminally ill. Incurable patients often were sent home to be looked after by their families, but most of them returned to the hospital to die. These hospitals were primarily cure-oriented. The staff was not trained to care for the dying. Given the general lack of skills and knowledge among the professional caregivers, symptom control and psychosocial care were often ineffective.

## A DEATH WITH NO DIGNITY

In 1981, I was working as a staff nurse in a "convalescent ward" of a general hospital where most patients were dying of cancer. These patients were sent to my ward from another acute hospital. The doctor came for ward rounds once a week.

I saw many patients die in physical and emotional distress. One night a patient pressed the help button every 15 minutes, asking for pain relief. I gave him all the prescribed medicine, but it didn't help him at all. He died a few days later, suffering till the end. It was a very frustrating experience for me. I felt that it had been my responsibility as a nurse to relieve this man's suffering, but I had not been able to do anything for him.

I shared my sense of failure with a pastoral counselor who visited the ward regularly. She told me that she had recently visited some hospices in England and the United States. Terminally ill people received very effective care in these hospice programs, and training courses were offered for the caregivers. This was the first time I had heard about hospice care. A few months later, I went to a hospice in England for training.

## THE FIRST TEAM

When I returned from England in 1982, I joined a hospital and set up a palliative care support team. This team provided the first palliative care service in Hong Kong. I was the nurse-coordinator and the only full-time member. A few professional colleagues who were interested in palliative care volunteered their support.

I visited dying patients throughout the hospital and worked with the ward staff to provide palliative care. Team members met regularly to discuss patient care and provide mutual support.

Initial response from other hospital staff members was not very positive. There were a lot of doubts about whether it was necessary to set up the palliative care team. Many staff members asked, "What more is there to be done for the dying?" More questions were asked when the service was in operation, especially about the use of strong narcotics and the time and attention we gave to psychological care.

A great deal of effort was spent on educating our colleagues through informal discussion in the clinical setting, as well as during inservice training programs. It took some time for the palliative care team to establish trust and credibility. Mutual support among the team members was especially important during this difficult process. Fortunately, the team members shared the same philosophy of patient care and were able to affirm and support each of us as we faced confrontations and challenges.

## THE BEGINNING OF PUBLIC AWARENESS

The team was functioning quietly in its small hospital until February, 1984, when a television crew produced a documentary program about our service. During the television interview, a patient talked openly about what he had gone through during his illness. This narrative included the pain of separation from his wife and children and how the palliative service had supported him and his family at a most difficult time.

After the program was telecast, we were overwhelmed by telephone calls from newspaper, radio, and television reporters asking for interviews. The mass media had a quick and powerful effect in publicizing palliative care. Patients and relatives called up to ask for help. Health care organizations and professional groups also requested lectures. This media-generated wave of interest marked the beginning of public education regarding hospice care in Hong Kong.

## FORMING A SOCIETY FOR PROMOTION OF
## HOSPICE CARE

There was still only one palliative care team in Hong Kong in 1985, and we were serving a very small number of patients. Because there was an obvious need for more palliative care programs, I met monthly with a few interested friends to explore the possibility of developing the needed additional programs. A year later we received financial support from the Keswick Foundation. This support enabled us to establish The Society for the Promotion of Hospice Care as a registered charity in Hong Kong.

It was a humble beginning. We started the Society in a tiny office inside a hospital, and for the first two years I was the only staff member. Because of our limited resources, it was still impossible to start hospice services at that time. We focused our efforts on education, in the belief that awareness and knowledge were crucial in developing hospice care. Not only did we organize educational services for health care programs, but we also undertook a wide range of activities to promote hospice care in the community. Lectures, courses, workshops, and exhibitions were organized in hospitals, professional training schools, and health care organizations.

One of the major difficulties in attempting to start hospice care in this Chinese society was the avoidance attitude toward death that has already been noted. For example, I was turned down by an estate manager when trying to rent an office as a base for promoting hospice care. His reason was that the neighbors would strongly object to having a death-tainted establishment in their locale. This attitude extended to some of the media as well. The producer of a television program contacted me for an interview. After receiving an accurate picture of hospice philosophy and practice, he said he would not air the interview. Why? "The audience would feel very upset to hear about death on a morning program."

Public education through the mass media and training programs for health care professionals brought about a change in the level of receptiveness toward the hospice approach. Over the years, the mass media have frequently reported on the hospice movement and the development of its services in Hong Kong. The death taboo was to some extent broken down through this open public discourse. This educational work has developed rapidly since 1986. The number of educational events increased from 47 in 1986 to 300 in 1994 (Chung, 1994). The philosophy, attitudes, and skills of hospice care were shared in these programs with the thousands of health care colleagues and members of the general public who attended each year.

## SETTING UP THE HOME CARE SERVICE AND THE INDEPENDENT HOSPICE

As more people heard about hospice care, we began to receive calls from terminally ill patients and their families. As noted, most terminally ill patients at that time were sent home to be cared for by their families, and returned to hospital very shortly before death. The majority of the Hong Kong population live in small flats, where living conditions are very cramped and almost no privacy exists. Most patients find it impossible to get a doctor to visit them at home. With this situation in mind, a hospice home care service was established in 1988. The team gradually expanded from one nurse to a team of eleven nurses in 1995. This team now provides care for approximately 100 patients at any one time.

While we were providing home hospice services we observed that many patients did not have the luxury of a residence in which they could be cared for comfortably. We started to appeal for donations to establish the first free-standing hospice in Hong Kong. In 1989, the government agreed to provide a site for the hospice. Through the generosity of many charitable trusts and donors, we succeeded in raising enough funds to cover the building costs of the hospice and the annual running costs for three years. It was planned that the hospice would seek full funding from the government after these first three years of operation.

The Hospice opened in June, 1992. It consist of a 26-bed inpatient unit, a home care service, a day care program, and facilities for education. The hospice was purpose-built and designed to provide a therapeutic environment and a homelike atmosphere. Efforts were made in the design to facilitate the comfort and safety of patients as well as efficiency of operation.

## RECRUITMENT AND TRAINING OF HOSPICE STAFF

One of the most important steps in ensuring quality care was to develop a strong hospice care team. The recruitment of nurses was done over a period of six months before the hospice opened, coinciding with a period when the hospitals were facing a particularly difficult time because of a nurse shortage. Unexpectedly, the response to the recruiting endeavor was surprisingly good. There were 300 applicants for 30 nursing posts. Many of the applicants had attended our hospice education programs, and had developed an understanding of hospice care (Chung, 1993).

We took into consideration LaGrande's (1980) proposed guidelines for hiring hospice staff. We were looking for the personal and professional qualities that were considered important in hospice work. These included:

- Analysis of job characteristics;
- Analysis of the motivation to serve others;
- Analysis of applicants' personality characteristics, especially the ability to relate well to others and show sensitivity to human needs;
- Applicants' history in handling intensely stressful events; and
- Goal-oriented work experience and qualifications.

To ensure quality care, we organized a four-week full-time training course for the nurses before the hospice accepted its first patient. Apart from teaching the skills of hospice care, the course also aimed at developing shared values and team spirit among the members of the clinical team. The course evaluation showed that all the nurses were aware of a substantial increase in their knowledge of various aspects of palliative care. They reproted that they benefitted most in the areas of communication and counseling skills, self-awareness, and understanding psychological aspect of death (Chung, 1992).

Careful selection and education of staff were key factors contributing to the success of the hospice service.

## THE SYSTEM OF OPERATION

The system of patient care is designed to enhance a patient-centered and individualized program. Deliberate efforts are made to reduce routine and nonessential tasks as much as possible.

A nursing care plan is worked out with each patient according to his or her individual needs. Quality assurance programs and regular inservice training sessions are organized to ensure a high standard of care.

Most of the referrals come from the public hospitals in which most patients with advanced cancer are treated. There is an increasing number of referrals for inpatient care, a trend that reflects physicians' heightened awareness and acceptance of the hospice service. Most patients referred for such care areq uite ill or have severe physical and/or psychological problems. There are also some inappropriate referrals for placement of patients.

Many patients with advanced cancer are still being discharged from acute hospitals without any home support. Although these patients are not in the terminal stage of illness, they would certainly benefit from the support of a hospice home care team. It is a priority to continue to promote the hospice home care service both to the professionals and the public.

Owing to the limited number of beds in the hospice, priority of admission is given to those whose physical symptoms and psychosocial problems are most intense, and to those who come in for respite or terminal care. The average length of stay in the hospice is around 15 days. The home care and day care service provide a continuum of care when patients are discharged from the hospice.

## THE VOLUNTEER PROGRAM

Like many other hospice programs throughout the world, the Hong Kong program benefits greatly from the services provided by volunteers. In our program, volunteers work closely with the professional team in providing care for patients and their families. In a hectic society with busy people, it is not easy to attract volunteers who can serve in a regular and consistent manner. However, there is a small group of dedicated volunteers who do work for the hospice on a regular basis, as well as a larger group who come on occasions when their help is especially needed.

We believe that careful selection, appropriate training, and supervision are factors crucial for the success of the volunteer program. Both a basic and an extended training course are offered to volunteers. The basic course prepares them to work on task-related jobs, while the extended course prepares them to work directly with patients and families.

## RELIGIOUS BELIEFS AND PRACTICES

There is much diversity of religious beliefs and practices in Hong Kong. Some people hold to a particular formal religion, but many others follow the traditional practice of worshiping their ancestors and many gods.

The Quiet Room of the hospice provides space and privacy for patients to pray or contemplate on their own. Bibles and prayer books of various religions are available for patients' use in the room. The hospice has also established a network with leaders of various religious and church groups whom we can ask to visit patients for spiritual support.

## HOSPICE ROLE IN PALLIATIVE EDUCATION

Attention to professional and public education was important in establishing Bradbury Hospice, Hong Kong's first such program. There has been not only a continuing but an increasing demand for palliative education, now that 10 other hospice units have been established in various hospitals.

The hospice plays an active role in palliative education. Courses and work-shops are organized regularly and receive enthusiastic response from professional carergivers. We are also invited to teach regularly in 10 medical and nursing schools in Hong Kong, and have organized training programs for the staff of several newly established hospice units.

There is an increasing number of requests for clinical placements for doctors, nurses, and social workers, both in the inpatient unit and the home care team. Starting from 1993, the Certificate Course in Hospice Nursing has been offered at Bradbury Hospice to provide systematic education in palliative nursing. Nurses had to go overseas for training before this course was offered locally. With the establishment of local educational programs, a larger number of health professionals in Hong Kong can prepare themselves to offer palliative care.

## DO CHINESE PATIENTS TALK ABOUT DEATH?

There is a common belief that Chinese are very reserved and prefer not to talk about death. Psychological intervention and open communication with patients about their disease are therefore considered to be inappropriate for Chinese patients. From his experience of working with Canadian Chinese, Tong (1994) reports that the cultural conflict between Western health professionals and Chinese families is one of the most controversial issues in serving Chinese palliative care patients. In Chinese culture, when there is a life-threatening situation, the family rarely hold open discussions in the presence of the patient. This practice conflicts with the current palliative care philosophy, which advocates openness and honesty toward patients when discussing their illness and impending death.

We faced similar situations in working with Chinese patients when we started our palliative care service in Hong Kong about 10 years ago. In practice, many doctors informed the family members about the poor prognosis, but did not tell the patient. The family members tried their best to hide the bad news from the patient. Although the family members were doing what they considered to be in the best interest of their loved ones, we often found that the dying patients felt helpless, isolated, and angry. The truth was kept from them, thereby excluding them from participating in many important decisions regarding their own lives.

From my experience of working with Chinese patients in Hong Kong, I am convinced that most patients want to talk about their impending death at some point during their terminal illness. However, many patients have been stopped by other people when they did express the desire to talk about death. Sensing an attitude of avoidance on the part of others, they would talk only to professional caregivers who had the courage, skills, and commitment to listen.

Chinese patients in general are more reserved and need more time to build up trust and to feel secure enough to talk about their impending death as compared with Westeners. It is therefore very important for hospice workers to be sensitive to the feelings of their patients. It is also important that they have the skills to facilitate the sharing and to respond therapeutically when a patient raises the subject of dying. In the case of patients and families who have chosen not to discuss death openly, it is important to respect and accept their ways of coping.

Since many patients and their families have difficulty in talking about their life-threatening situations, professional caregivers often have a major role in facilitating understanding and communication between patient and family. With the support of professional caregivers, the patient and the family are encouraged to communicate openly, after mutual support, and settle unfinished business before the patient dies. In situations where the family is unwilling to communicate openly with the patient, the professional caregivers who offer to listen and support can minimize the feelings of isolation and loneliness.

Hospice care has initiated a change from the long-established practice of not telling patients their prognoses, to one which respects the patients' right to know and which facilitates open communication. This new approach has produced positive results among Chinese patients. We have learned from our experience that many Chinese patients do talk about their impending death if given the permission. The attitudes and reactions of Chinese patients toward death are areas which need systematic research and evaluation.

## CONCLUSION

The hospice movement has developed rapidly in Hong Kong over the past decade. We have witnessed a growing interest in palliative care among health care professionals and the general public. A freestanding hospice has been established and palliative care services have been established in various hospitals to provide better care for the dying. After three years of operation that relied entirely on donations, the management of the Bradbury Hospice was transferred to Hospital Authority of Hong Kong in 1995.

All these developments attest to an increasing awareness of the needs of the terminally ill in our society. The new challenge for us is to facilitate the development of hospice care in hospitals and the community. We hope that we can continue to promote the philosophy of hospice care and improve the quality of life for the terminally ill in Hong Kong by sharing our ideas and knowledge through education and clinical care.

## REFERENCES

Chung, L. (1992). *Report on hospice nursing course*. Unpublished manuscript.
Chung, L. (1993). Setting up a nursing service in a new hospice: A Hong Kong experience. *Asian Journal of Nursing Studies, 1*, 46–51.
Chung, L. (1994). *Statistical report on hospice education programs*. Unpublished manuscript.
LaGrande, L. E. (1980). Reducing burnout in the hospice and the death education movement. *Death Education, 4*, 61–75.
Tong, K. L. (1994). The Chinese palliative patient and family in North America: A cultural perspective. *Journal of Palliative Care, 10*, 26–28.

**20**

# Development of Palliative Care in India

## G. L. Burn

Dr. Jan Stjernsward, the chief of the Cancer and Palliative Care unit of the World Health Organization, has made palliative care a priority for developing countries as part of WHO's National Cancer Control Programs. In newly industralized countries, 80% of the cancer patients are first diagnosed in the terminal phase of their illness, when palliative care is the only humane and pragmatic solution. It is vital to make palliative care available to the entire public. Stjernsward (1993) reports that only an estimated 5–10% of cancer resources are spent on 90% of the world's cancer population. Very often, these precious resources are spent on expensive but inappropriate cancer therapy where there is no hope of cure, but where there could be a hope of relief for suffering.

We can look at the example of India to identify some of the issues involved in establishing palliative care programs in developing countries. It is easy for experts in palliative care in the Western world to describe and promote the correct use of oral morphine, but it is a different matter in a country where the use of morphine is not legal in several states. Alternative drugs, such as buprenorphine, may or may not be available. Often, the cost of such drugs is prohibitive to the majority of patients who could benefit from them.

There are also bureaucratic hoops that one must jump through. These include licenses to prescribe, hold, and dispense morphine. Often morphine can be prescribed only by a hospital, and not by a community physician. Furthermore,

215

some hospitals insist that only inpatients can have morphine. This dictum forces a choice between potentially dying pain-free in a hospital, separated from family and home, or dying at home in pain. Patients and caregivers often choose the former to try to avoid intolerable suffering, as well as possible abandonment by both health care professionals and family/informal caregivers.

The WHO is striving to ensure that morphine is made available when needed to relieve the suffering of terminally ill cancer sufferers (Stjernsward, Koroltchouk, & Teoh, 1992; World Health Organization [WHO], 1994). Government officials, doctors, and the public are afraid of addiction in the patient, and also afraid that widespread abuse of morphine might occur via theft of the drug from pharmacies or patients. There is also concern that relatives may abuse the drugs. Respiratory depression and tolerance leading to ever-escalating doses is also feared. In a word, morphine is seen as synonymous with death. It is vital that the WHO "process triangle" is in place—i.e., drug availability, government policy, and education—if correct use of the drug is to be achieved.

Poverty, illiteracy, ignorance of the warning signs of disease, long distances from the hospital, and fear and stigma associated with cancer all compound the problem from the patients' point of view and interfere with their seeking early referral (Burn, 1994a). Lack of education regarding the use of oral morphine, fears of addiction and respiratory depression, and difficulties in actually acquiring the drug hamper its use on the part of health care professionals. Working conditions in India and other developing countries often are extremely difficult. Wards are overcrowded. Not infrequently, patients must sleep on the floor. Doctors outnumber nurses 3 : 1 in India, and the patient-nurse ratio can be in the range of 60–80 : 1. These considerations make it imperative that palliative care is achieved in the community and that the patients and their families are empowered to receive and deliver care at home. This initiative will need to come from health care professionals, which means that they, in turn, must be knowledgeable and confident in their delivery of palliative care.

## CANCER RELIEF INDIA

Cancer Relief India (CRI) is a small United Kingdom-based charity that was formed in 1990 with the aim of addressing the issue of education. The director has been involved since that time in initiatives to educate doctors and nurses in palliative care. This activity has involved awareness-raising programs in India for both the public and professionals. Individualized training programs in palliative care have also been provided in the UK.

The program includes two different clinical attachments, primarily in community and hospital settings, but also in designated inpatient palliative care units. Instruction is also given in the theory of palliative care. Because education and coverage (or dissemination) are seen as the cornerstones of care, the course also includes teaching and communications skills as well as the management of change. It is expected that the knowledge gained through this course will be shared with others upon the caregivers' return home, thus creating a cascade effect.

A positive outcome from one of the courses has been the setting up of the first hospital-based palliative care team in India. This service is based in a government hospital in Calicut under the direction of two physicians who have completed the UK course. They have inspired their colleagues to work collaboratively and have also encouraged a team of about 20 volunteers to help them. The costs of the clinic are funded in part by CRI. The team works on a referral basis. Referring consultants keep their own patients, but use the expertise of the team for advice on symptom management. The team is also involved in education programs with students and postgraduates and is very keen to have doctors and nurses working a clinical attachment so that they, in turn, can develop their skills and teach others.

The WHO consider that this clinic in Calicut is a model for developing countries. It sees 50 to 60 patients per day, and in two years has served more than a thousand new patients. There are no inpatient designated beds for this service. The team works in a collaborative manner that is beneficial for professional and patient alike. Meanwhile, Varanasi, a nurse in North India, having completed the UK course, has written a booklet on palliative care for the population at large, and in the local language. He has also been instrumental in the foundation of a rural palliative care center (Burn, 1993, 1994, 1995).

Collectively, these individual initiatives have raised the profile of palliative care in India and encouraged larger concerns to take an interest. The first hospice in India was started in the mid-1980s. Palliative care has now spread to the hospital and community. An exciting development that will soon be in operation is the establishment of a palliative care unit with a designated education center that will affirm the importance of theory and practice working in unison, if the WHO goal of palliative care for all by the year 2000 is to be achieved.

# REFERENCES

Burn, G. L. (1993). *Reports of Visits to India*. London: Cancer Relief Macmillan Fund.

Burn, G. L. (1994a). Palliative care in India. *Cancer Care, 1*, 1–3.

Burn, G.L. (1994b). *Reports of visits to India*. London: Cancer Relief Macmillan Fund.

Burn, G.L. (1995). *Reports of visits to India*. London: Cancer Relief Macmillan Fund.

Stjernsward, J. (1993). Palliative medicine: A global perspective. In D. D. Hanks &N. MacDonald (Eds.), *Oxford textbook of palliative medicine* (pp. 805–816), Oxford: Oxford University Press.

Stjernsward, J., Koroltchouk, V., & Teoh, N. (1992). National policies for cancer pain relief and palliative care. *Palliative Medicine, 6,* 273–276.

World Health Organization (1994). Cancer pain relief: A guide to opioid availability (2nd edition). In *Palliative cancer care: Pain relief and management of other symptoms.* Geneva: World Health Organization, pp. 41–59.

# 21

# Hospice Care in Japan

Mitsuaki Sakonji, M. D., Chise Shimizu,
Yae Shingo, Eitaka Tauboi, M. D.

---

## INTRODUCTION

The first hospice in Japan was Seirei Mikatagahara Hospice in Hamamatsu City, which was established in 1981. Since that time, several other hospice programs have been established throughout Japan. In 1990, the Ministry of Health and Welfare (MOW) included care provided for terminally ill patients in Palliative Care Unit (PCUs) in the health insurance system. People eligible for care in PCUs are restricted to those with terminal cancer or progressed AIDS. The established standards for PCUs are quite detailed (Table 21.1).

In Japan, all people belong to the national health care system, and are able to receive basically the same level of treatment at any facility for a relatively small fee. This health insurance system has been the primary factor in providing the Japanese with the world's longest lifespan. Because of the increase in the average length of life, Japan is also developing a graying population at an exceptional rate. This growth of the elder population is affecting public demand for care. Request for medical treatment in some areas is changing from a focus on quantity to concerns about quality. Even in the case of terminal cancer care, we are receiving more requests regarding quality of life (QOL) treatment. We are also receiving requests from the general population for an increase in hospice programs.

As of November 1995, there were only 20 PCU facilities recognized by the MOW. These facilities had a total of 392 beds, or 0.03 % of total hospital beds

**TABLE 21.1 Standards for Establishment of Palliative Care Unit (MOW)**

1. Patients limited to cases with terminally malignant tumors or Acquired Immune Deficiency Syndrome, and must be admitted for cumulative care.
2. The hospital concerned must provide one nurse for each 1.5 patients per ward.
3. The issue of whether the health diagnosis emolument at the hospital concerned uses a new nursing system or standard nursing system should be resolved.
4. Must provide the number of doctors required by law.
5. Must provide a full-time physician on hand for palliative care.
6. An actual floor space of the ward of at least $30\,m^2$ per patient, not counting pillar or wall space. Not less than $8\,m^2$ per patient per room.
7. About 50% of the rooms in the ward should be private.
8. A waiting room, kitchen, consultation room, and lounge hall should be provided.
9. Special medical treatment environment rooms for patients who must pay an additional fee to be less than 50% of the total.
10. A judgement committee should be established to evaluate the patient's condition and decide on release.

*Source*: Health Insurance Law, Japanese MOW (#40, 199).

available (Table 21.2). There were an additional 15 facilities that did not belong to the Japanese Hospice-PCU Contact Conference Organization. However, since the PCU facilities in these hospitals are counted as "regular beds" by the Japanese health care system, we cannot know exactly how many special care units or beds they have.

In 1994, there were about 880,000 deaths in Japan, of which about 26%, or 240,000, occurred due to malignant neoplasms, including leukemia. According to the AIDS Surveillance Report by the MOW, the cumulative total cases of AIDS as of 1994 was 1,845 HIV-positive cases, with 404 fully developed cases.

These figures make it clear that the number of PCUs available in Japan today is not enough to provide for the number of patients in need. An additional problem is that in Japan, the term PCU often is thought of as only a process for relieving pain, and thus as a sort of negative euthanasia. However, there is a difference of nuance between that idea and the idea of hospice care, which helps the patients experience a high quality of life during the time they have left. Therefore, we need enlightenment on hospice care. The hope is that the understanding of the true meaning of hospice care, and an increase in facilities available, will make possible a greater response to citizen demands, and increases in the number of volunteers.

## HOSPICE CARE IN TSUBOI HOSPITAL

Tsuboi Cancer Center Hospital is located in Kohriyama City, Fukushima Prefecture. In 1977, the hospital was established as an attached facility of the Jizankai

TABLE 21.2 Establishment of Palliative Care Units (As of November 1995)

| Name of Hospital | Number of PCU beds/ Total beds | Date of MOW Approval |
|---|---|---|
| Seirei Mikatagahara Hospital | 27/758 | 90.04.25 |
| Yodogawa Christian Hospital | 23/600 | 90.04.25 |
| Salvation Army Kiyose Hospital | 30/195 | 90.05.29 |
| Fukuoka Kameyama Eikô Hospital | 24/128 | 90.08.29 |
| Jizankai Medical Foundation Tsuboi Hospital | 18/312 | 90.11.29 |
| Ageo Kôsei Hospital | 13/120 | 92.02.25 |
| National Cancer Center Higashi Hospital | 25/425 | 92.07.01 |
| Toyama Prefectual Chûô Hospital | 15/800 | 93.02.25 |
| Nagaoka Nishi Hospital | 22/136 | 93.03.12 |
| Higashi Sapporo Hospital | 28/250 | 93.09.01 |
| Kobe Adventist Hospital | 8/116 | 93.09.29 |
| Peace House | 22/22 | 94.02.01 |
| Nishi Gunma Hospital | 24/480 | 94.07.01 |
| National Medical Care Home St. John's Sakuramachi Hospital | 20/276 | 94.08.01 |
| Jesuit Mental Institute Hospital | 15/87 | 94.11.01 |
| Rokkô Hospital | 23/178 | 94.12.01 |
| Ishikawa Prefecture Saiseikai Kanazawa Hospital | 28/260 | 95.01.01 |
| Yokohama Kôsei Hospital | 12/86 | 95.02.01 |
| Mt Olive Hospital | 7/343 | 95.06.01 |
| Nihon Baptist Hospital | 8/155 | 95.09.01 |

Source: Turn of approval by Minister of MOW; Official Garette of Japanese Government.

Medical Research Center Foundation. The purpose of the Foundation is research into educational activities, and activities necessary for cancer prevention and early diagnosis; development of high standards for medical personnel working with cancer; and arrangement of special medical treatment facilities. Therefore, Tsuboi Hospital aimed at specialization in cancer research and care from the beginning. As such, the basic policies of management are as follows: (1) Enlightenment or diffusion of cancer knowledge through lectures, television programs, or other educational means; (2) Completion of a medical examination system for early diagnosis and treatment of cancer; (3) Training of staff to improve diagnosis and provide joint cancer treatment and care; and (4) Perfection of hospice care to improve the quality of life of terminal cancer patients.

Today, Tsuboi Hospital has a total of 312 beds, with 83% of the patients undergoing treatment for malignant neoplasm. Some patients are in the terminal cancer stage when they enter the program. When the hospital first opened, the main form of care for terminal patients was the visiting nurse system. However, if the patient's residence was far from the hospital or the care-giver was becoming exhaused, the patient would be moved into the hospital. When the patients were at home, they were surrounded by their family and friends, so their QOL was rather good. But when they came to the hospital they began to share their life with others who had undergone operations, or were going through chemotherapy and other types of treatment, so oftentimes their QOL degenerated.

After some time, there was a request from the nursing section to create beds for hospice-type care for these patients. As a result, in June 1990, we remodeled a 56-bed ward and reopened it as a hospice ward with 18 beds. In December of that same year, the Ministry of Health and Welfare recognized the ward as a palliative care unit.

The hospice has 10 private rooms and two four-bed rooms, 14 nurses, one specialist doctor, two assistant nurses, one office worker, and one caseworker. They also utilize volunteers to help with spcial events, visit patients, take care of room plants and flowers, and assist with other social concerns. The hospice at Tsuboi Hospital is modeled on the Saint Francis Hospice in Hawaii. In 1988, we sent some nurses to Saint Francis for research and study, and have sent about 10 staff members every year since.

The Tsuboi Hospice is not related to any particular religious organization, and places no limit on the amount of religious activity which believers might practice in their rooms. There are also few rules limiting alcohol or tobacco. Patients may also keep pets with them, if they so choose. The rules concerning visiting hours by family and friends are also rather free. Thus all patients are generally free to pursue their daily lives, so long as they do not disturb other patients.

Since Tsuboi Hospital's hospice program is mainly a home-care program, the hospice ward is primarily for patients who for some reason cannot receive home care. The management framework is based on the concept of using home care, inpatient care, and outpatient day care in an organically related manner (Figure 21.1). The actual hospice management and coordination is provided by the nursing stuff and coordinator. The Foundation director and the chairman of the hospital are advisors to the hospice management.

Between 1989 and 1994, 236 patients used the hospice care facilities at Tsuboi Hospital. These included 49 home care patients and 187 were inpatients (Figure 21.2). The ages of the hospice patients ranged from 33 to 94, with an average age of 64.8. The largest number of men were aged 71–80, and the largest number of women were aged 61–70 (Figure 21.3). The major causes of death for one-third of the men was lung and gastric cancer, while for women, there was no particularly salient characteristic (Figure 21.4).

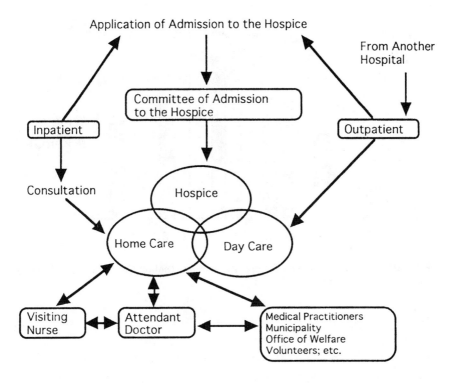

FIGURE 21.1 The System of Hospice Care at Tsuboi Cancer Center Hospital

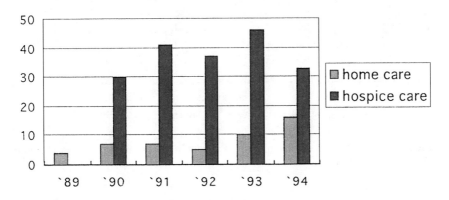

FIGURE 21.2 Number of Hospice Care Patients in Tsuboi Cancer Center Hospital Hospice

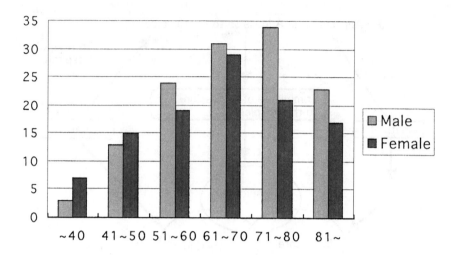

FIGURE 21.3 Age of Hospice Care Patients in Tsuboi Cancer Center Hospital Hospice (1989–1994)

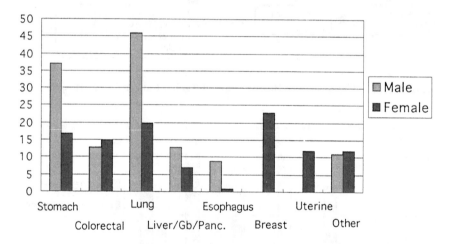

FIGURE 21.4 Diseases of Hospice Care Patients in Tsuboi Cancer Center Hospital Hospice (1989–1994)

The percentage of patients who were informed of their condition was 61% (Figure 21.5). However, the yearly rate of patients informed has continued to increase, and was over 80% in 1994 (Figure 21.6).

Length of time spent in home care was an average of 86 days, with the longest being 764 days. Average inpatient stay was 48.3 days, with the longest being 405

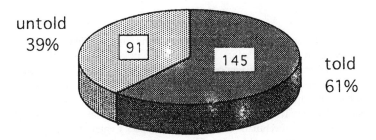

untold
39%

told
61%

FIGURE 21.5 Percentage of Patients Who Were Told About Their Disease in Tsuboi Cancer Center Hospital Hospice (1989–1994)

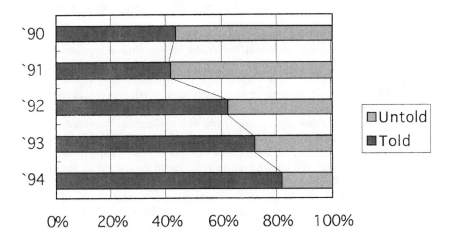

FIGURE 21.6 Yearly Rate of Patients Told About Their Disease in Tsuboi Cancer Center Hospital Hospice

days. In 49 cases of home care, 13 patients died at home, and the other 36 died after being moved to the hospice.

## THREE INFLUENTIAL CASES

Here, I would like to introduce three cases that left an especially strong impression.

# Case Study I

A 33-year-old junior high school teacher was living a normal life with her husband and two children. One year before, she began to complain of pain in her chest. The medical university hospital diagnosed her condition as Ewing's sarcoma of the chest wall. She underwent an operation and was placed on chemotherapy treatment. Later, she suffered a relapse of sarcoma, accompanied by a pleurisy and multiple spread of metastasized bone. The resultant pain created difficulty in breathing and general functioning, and she eventually entered Tsuboi Cancer Center Hospital.

The patient was completely aware of her condition, and requested relief from the difficulty in breathing as well as the pain. She also decided to utilize hospice care. A puncture was created to remove the pleural effusion responsible for the difficulty in breathing. To control pain, a radiotherapy program with Lineac injection into the affected areas was started. Also, in an effort to slow the progression of the sarcoma as much as possible, a program of oral etoposide was utilized to limit side effects and adverse reactions. At the same time, she was being given morphine sulfate for general pain control.

When the patient entered the hospital, she was unable to turn over by herself. Within one month she was able to walk to the toilet, and her physical appearance was improved. At two months postadmission, with the aid of a walker, she was able to join other patients and volunteer workers for a picnic lunch near the hospital. She also had an interest in crafts, and sometime went out with relatives or volunteers to purchase craft materials.

She also planned to take part in a family trip with her husband and children. She brought a sewing machine to her room and made carrying bags for the children to use on the trip. At five months postadmission she was able to make the trip (lasting two nights and three days). The husband took a videotape of the trip, which showed a happy and joyful family. She was a believer in Christianity, but was not baptized. Therefore, after the trip she underwent baptism in her room. At six months postadmission she took a turn for the worse and died with her family in attendance. She knew that she didn't have much time left, but she maintained her purposes of daily life. Every time I saw her, I could see in her face that she was telling us how important hospice care is for giving us precious time to live. After she died, I had a few chances to see her husband. He told me that it was a wonderful thing for her family that she was able to spend time in the hospice during her last six months.

# Case Study II

An 83-year-old man who had undergone a rectal cancer operation three years previously entered an outpatient program at Tsuboi Hospital because of pain in the left femoral and the problem of urgency. Investigation showed a recurrence of the pelvic tumor, which was resulting in pressure on the bladder and nerve. Taking into consideration his age and general condition, the patient decided on hospice care rather than an operation.

Soon after entering the hospice inpatient program, he was put on 50 mg diclonac sodium suppository twice a day to control pain. Since this medication soon proved to be insufficient, he was put on a daily oral dose of 40 mg morphine sulfate. This addressed the pain problem and also helped to clear up the urgency. As a result, he was able to go on an outpatient hospice program, during which he received weekly home visits from the nursing staff; the doctor would visit him once a month.

He and his wife were active in his hobby of making pottery. When I visited him, he showed me many of the cups and big plates that he has made, and I came to realize how difficult it is to make the beautiful patterns and color combinations. He presented me with one of his favorite pieces, a vase with a butterfly design as a memorial, which I still proudly display in the entrance to my house.

At seven months postadmission his pain worsened—he had by now been put on 120 mg morphine a day—so his family wanted him to enter the hospice inpatient program. At that time, he was in pain and suffered paralysis in both legs. He also was in a weakened condition from lack of proper diet. He was unable to take oral doses of morphine, which required that it be added to a drip-infusion water supply. The patient requested that only painkillers be given during the final days. In respect of his wishes, the hospice did not give him any additional dietary supplements, and he died peacefully.

The seven months the patient spent at his own home were very fulfilling for him and his wife, and his memory is kept alive through the works of art he made that remain with his family and friends, including me.

## Case Study III

A 49-year-old priest had undergone a rectal cancer operation. At that time, the cancer had already showed signs of advancing to the liver. He received a detailed explanation of his illness.

Seven months after the operation, he began showing symptoms of stomach pressure and came to Tsuboi Hospital for testing. He was informed that he had an accumulation of ascites, and was admitted in an effort to control the situation. He was given an abdominal puncture to remove the ascites, and was prescribed an oral diuretic. Diclonac sodium suppository was used to control stomach pain. There was improvement in the symptom of stomach pressure, and the patient wanted to return home under the hospice outpatient program.

On day 11, he returned to his home. He had a 12-year-old daughter and an 8-year-old son. However, since both children were in school, his wife was given the task of home care. He was unable to maintain a proper diet, but refused nutrition supplement through drip infusion. His wife made foods that he could eat available to him as much as possible.

The patient was on a home nurse visiting program with visits scheduled every two days, and had three episodes of hospice day care in order to remove the ascites. At 24 days postadmission to the hospice program, the stomach pressure symptoms began to increase and he was readmitted as an inpatient. By that time, the stomach pain was more intense.

After entering the hospice, he was put on a drip infusion, and given morphine suppositories for pain. He also underwent abdominal puncture again for removal of ascites. He wanted to return home again, and did so five hours after admittance, after which the nurses began a daily visit program. His level of consciousness began to weaken, and he died at 31 days after his primary admittance to Tsuboi Hospital.

The time that he stayed at home was only 21 days. During that time, most of his concern was about his children's future. He also most likely wanted to show his children positive attitudes toward life and death, both as a father and a priest. In the beginning, the children were very afraid of death, and avoided contact with their father. Soon, though, they were able to accept their father's imminent death and they were able to give positive aid to him by supporting their mother and helping to take care of him themselves.

The sadness of the bereaved family is hard to imagine, but this experience was able to leave them with a faith in the wonderfullness of life which they were able to carry forward in their hearts.

I have introduced three cases which we have experienced, but they are only samples taken from many such cases, each of which has its own story. Every time we meet a person who is attempting to deal with terminal cancer, we learn more about life. And everything that we learn is a very precious experience, and I believe that this stock of experience will help us to improve future hospice care.

## DISCUSSION

The Japanese are guaranteed religious freedom by the Constitution. Therefore, they are free to choose any religion, and the depth of belief depends on the person. In 20 of the PCUs established by the MOW (see Table 21.2), nine were affiliated with Christian institutions, and one with a Buddhist organization. The others, including Tsuboi Hospice, are not directly related to any particular religious organization or group.

Perhaps the background of hospital development in Japan is one reason for the lack of connection between the hospices and religious organizations. Hospitals in Japan are mainly established by individual doctors as an expansion of their clinical facilities; established by the prefectural government; or are designated as national hospitals. There are a few hospitals with characteristics similar to America or Europe, such as those established by charity groups or monasteries.

The foundation of the Japanese way of thinking was greatly influenced by Confucianism. The primary resource document is *The Analects*, written by Confucius around 500 B.C. Confucianism, mixed with the indigenous Japanese religion and customs, has created a unique view of life among the Japanese. In Japan we have the phrase: "Do my best and leave the rest to Providence." This Japanese point of view is somewhat different than that of the Christian nations, whose people often believe that when things don't work out, no matter how hard they try, they should accept it as God's will. The Japanese people often feel that even though they may not succeed, they should always make their best effort. If we do not make such effort, other people will blame us for giving up too soon or not trying enough.

This attitude carries over into the experience of terminal illness. Patients who are in the terminal stage of cancer tell us that they have fought with cancer enough, and they want to spend the rest of their life peacefully in the hospice. When family or friends hear such talk, they urge the patient to fight more, and at times try to prevent the patient from entering the hospice.

It is a Japanese characteristic to try to shield those close to us from any pain or trouble because of sympathy for family and friends. Families sometimes ask the doctor not to tell patients of their condition. At times, even when the doctor thinks it best to talk frankly with the patient, the family will request that he not do so. This emotional background is one reason for the traditionally low rate of patient-informing in Japan.

In 1994, a MOW social economic research survey showed that 93.8% of families who had a member die from cancer received an explanation from doctor (Figure 21.7); 20.2% of the patients were informed themselves; 43.8% guessed that they had the disease; and 28.8% never knew of their condition (Figure 21.8). Thus, we can see there is a big gap between the family members who knew the situation and the patients themslves.

Earlier there were many inpatients in our hospice who were not informed of their disease. But, as I said before, the rate of patient-informing is increasing every year (see Figure 21.6), and our doctors favor the approach of fighting the cancer

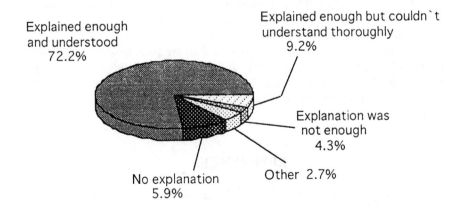

Explained enough and understood 72.2%

Explained enough but couldn`t understand thoroughly 9.2%

Explanation was not enough 4.3%

No explanation 5.9%

Other 2.7%

FIGURE 21.7 Explanation to the Family About the Therapeutic Plan for Cancer Patients (Investigation of the movement of population in Japan, 1994. By Japanese Ministry of Health and Welfare)

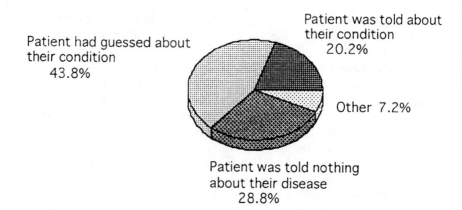

Patient had guessed about their condition 43.8%

Patient was told about their condition 20.2%

Other 7.2%

Patient was told nothing about their disease 28.8%

FIGURE 21.8 Percentage of Patients Told or who Had Guessed About Their Disease (Investigation of the movement of population in Japan, 1994. By Japanese Ministry of Health and Welfare)

with the knowledge of the patient. In the future, the reformation of doctors' views may encourage them to persuade families to tell the patient the truth.

According to a survey from the National Cancer Center (1988), 60.7% of those questioned think that a hospice is the last stop before death, and 41.2% think the patients have no chance of recovery. So there is a rather dark image of hospice programs among the general population, and there are many who still think of a hospice as simply a place to go to die. To spread hospice care, we need to change this conception. Toward that goal, those of us who deal with hospice care must make much more effort at enlightenment activities to create an understanding of the characteristics and meaning of the program.

While patients are fighting the disease and trying to understand their own illness, relapse and transition occurs, and when entering the terminal stage patients should be able to choose hospice or home care by their own will. Providing a good system and developing facilities to allow for such choicemaking is the task for Japan today.

## REFERENCES

Hinohara, S., & Yamamoto, S. (Eds.) (1988). *Thanatology* (Vol. 1). Tokyo: Gijutsu.

Honda, K. (1994). Relations with patients and families in the hospice ward. *Nurse Data, 15,* 42–46.

National Cancer Center Hospital (1988). In K. Hiraga (Ed.) (1991), *Terminal medical care.* Osaka: Saishin Igakusha.

Ministry of Health and Welfare of Japan (Ed.) (1995). *White paper on public welfare at 1994.* Tokyo: Public Welfare Problems Research Foundation.

Tsuboi, E., & Shinjo, Y. (1993). Hospice and home care in Tsuboi Hospital. *The Journal of Public Health Practice, 57,* 618–622.

*Near East*

# 22

# Hospice and Palliative Care Services in Israel

## Alexander Waller, MD

### Historical Background

The foundations of the modern hospice movement in Israel were probably laid during the same period in the Middle Ages when Christian hospices began to flourish along the routes taken by Crusaders and Christian pilgrims to the Holy Land. In the Christian hospices of that period, travelers who came from far away found bed and board and—if ill or dying—appropriate care. The needy of the neighborhood received the same consideration.

During that same period, the institution of the *hekdesh* was evolving in the Jewish Diaspora throughout Europe. The word "hekdesh" signifies consecrated property, specifically property set aside for charitable purposes or for the fulfillment of *mitzvoth* (religiously prescribed deeds). By the Middle Ages, the word had come to designate a communal shelter and infirmary for wayfarers, the destitute, and the sick. The *hekdesh* was generally administered by a local association (*hevrah*). This was most commonly the *hevret bikkur cholim* (association of visitors to the sick) or *hevrat kadishe* (burial society), under the supervision of the Jewish community. The *gebbel* or *beadle* of the association was often a local merchant, and his job was to visit the *hekdesh* at least daily, and supervise the work of the doctors and attendants there.

Since most sick people during the Middle Ages were cared for at home, the *hekdesh* served mainly those who were without family or who were transients passing through the community, such as peddlers and journeying scholars. The emphasis on care of suffering travelers—whether their journey be physical or metaphysical—has persisted in nearly all hospice movements, of whatever religious persuasion, until the present. Thus, when Israel was still part of the Ottoman Empire, the Turks constructed a series of caravanserais (*hans*). The distance between any two of them was the distance which could be covered during a day's journey by camel. Those among the wayfarers who were ill or dying could be housed and receive care in the *hans*. The beautiful Han El-Umdan in St. Jane d'Acre is an example of one of these institutions.

## THE BEGINNINGS OF THE MODERN HOSPICE MOVEMENT IN ISRAEL: THE TEL HASHOMER HOSPICE

Modern hospice care in Israel had its beginnings in 1981, when Dr. Marian Rabinowitz, Chairman of the Department of Geriatrics at Chiam Sheba Medical Center, Tel Hashomer, and members of the Israeli Cancer Society decided to address the deficiencies they saw in the care of patients with advanced disease and of their families. To learn more about how care was provided to that patient population in other settings, Dr. Rabinovitz traveled to Germany and also to England, where he visited Dr. Cicely Saunders at St. Christopher's Hospice. Returning to Israel, he set up a group including physicians, nurses, a social worker, and a clinical psychologist to lay the groundwork for Israel's first hospice.

In March, 1983, Israel's first hospice, Tel Hashomer Hospice, was opened as an independent unit attached to Chaim Sheba Medical Center, the largest general hospital in the country. The aim of Tel Hashomer Hospice was, and remains, to give the best quality of life to patients with terminal cancer and to their families. From the outset Tel Hashomer Hospice has been a joint project of the Israel Cancer Society, the Ministry of Health, and the General Sick Fund. Each of the participating agencies provide an equal share of the operating costs, so that no direct fees are levied on the patients or their families. Administrative responsibility for Tel Hashomer Hospice resides in the Israeli Cancer Society.

At the time of its opening, Tel Hashomer Hospice had 25 beds, including two standby beds kep available for patients who needed readmission. The first medical director was Dr. Marian Rabinovitz, and the first head nurse was Mrs. Dvora Goren. Subsequently, medical directors came from the Geriatric Department of the Chaim Sheba Medical Center and worked on a rotating basis for approximately six months each. Evening and night shifts were covered by physicians on duty from the Geriatric Department. The development of Tel Hashomer Hospice is most conveniently described using the schema of Olsen (1988).

## THE PIONEERING PERIOD: 1983–1986

At the time that Tel Hashomer Hospice opened its doors, there was no practical experience in Israel in any field of palliative care. Dvora Goren read what books and papers about hospice that she was able to obtain (most of them from St. Christopher's Hospice). Books and periodicals on hospice care were scarce at that time, however, and the operation of an interdisciplinary team was undefined. For the most part, it was necessary to discover and invent everything from the beginning. Nonetheless, the general atmosphere among the staff was one of vocation, enthusiasm, and dedication, along with uncertainty about the most appropriate way to give support to the patient and the family.

The prevailing atmosphere resulted in perhaps too many meetings and too much talk, without genuine communication. Nonetheless, from the beginning, we did a lot of teaching. We held conferences and workshops. We promoted the concepts of hospice and palliative care on the general wards of hospitals and in the community. Education was also part of the admission procedure to hospice. The request for admission had to be presented to our admissions committee by the patient's own primary physician, nurse, and/or social worker. This admission request became an excellent occasion for medical professionals from outside the hospice to see the facility and learn about supportive care.

The pioneering period of Tel Hashomer Hospice started to draw to a close as we consolidated our initial experiences and compared it with the experiences of others. Our head nurse, Dvora Goren, visited the Royal Marsden Hospital and had the opportunity to learn from the experiences of Dr. Lamerton. I visited the St. Francis Hospice in Romford-Essex to learn from Dr. Anthony Smith, then medical director there, and visited also St. Christopher's Hospice to learn from Cicely Saunders, Mary Baines, and Tony O'Brien. The many things we learned in England helped us enormously in our routine work when we returned to Israel.

## THE TRANSITIONAL PERIOD: 1986–1992

As the Tel Hashomer Hospice matured, its administrative framework became firmer, and the time inevitably came when it was necessary to look at issues associated with financial accountability and solvency. This change from a free-wheeling, pioneering mission to a more stable structure produced tension between members of the team. Staff meetings were very stormy. Nonetheless, we continued to extend our services and carry out our teaching mission.

In 1989, I became medical director of the Tel Hashomer Hospice on a permanent basis, ending the system of rotating directorship and enabling more consistent policies and practices. During this period, with funding from the Israeli
Cancer Society, we established a home care hospice for an average daily census of
25 patients and their families living within a 20-kilometer radius of our inpatient
facility. We also began providing practical palliative care experience within the
hospice to medical students in the third and sixth year of their studies, to
oncology nurses and nursing students, and to social work students from Tel Aviv
University. We began to write about our experience and to present our findings
at international congresses and in foreign medical and nursing journals. We were
fortunate to have frequent visits from Dr. Anthony Smith, by then the Director of
Studies at St. Christopher's Hospice, and from other distinguished guests from
abroad, and we continued to benefit from the advice of Dr. Cicely Saunders.

## STABILIZATION: 1992–1995

This third period in the development of the Tel Hashomer Hospice has seen a
gradual accommodation between our ideals of the optimum support for the
patient with advanced cancer and the available resources.

The number of inpatient beds was reduced from 25 to 18 to preserve a nurse-
to-patient ration of 0.9. The role of each profession in the interdisciplinary team
has become clearer, and leadership has been better defined and understood.
Within the hospice itself, we have established a training center for nurses as well
as training for our volunteers. Our liaison nurse provides nursing consultation in
palliative care to hospitals and community-based doctors. Our participation in
international meetings has increased, as has our contribution to the international
medical literature on palliative care. To date we have published more than 15
papers in the medical literature, here and abroad. A comprehensive handbook
reflecting our experience in caring for over five thousand patients with advanced
cancer has been published (Wailer & Caroline, 1996).

Staffing to carry out our activities—the care of 18 patients and 25 home
hospice patients, the work of a liaison nurse, and the training center for nurses,
with medical and social work components—is as follows (Table 22.1).

With all the experience gained during the earlier periods of development, the
atmosphere in Tel Hashomer Hospice became one of professionalism and calm
assurance, and teamwork proceeded more smoothly and efficiently.

## FUTURE CHALLENGES FOR TEL HASHOMER HOSPICE

Our goals for the near future in the Tel Hashomer Hospice include the following:

TABLE 22.1 Staffing Pattern: Tel Hashomer Hospice

| Pole | Number of Full-Time Equivalent Positions |
| --- | --- |
| Physicians | 2.5 |
| Registered Nurses | 18.5 |
| Nursing Aides | 1.5 |
| Social Workers | 1.25 |
| Clinical Psychologist | 0.3 |
| Occupational Therapist | 0.3 |
| Secretary | 1.6 |
| Administrative Director | 0.5 |
| Volunteers | 20.0 |

- To conduct well-designed evaluation studies of our work;
- To enlarge our training center and to strengthen its medical and social work components;
- To provide day care for outpatients;
- To open an outpatient clinic for consultation and followup; and
- To establish a hospital support team.

## THE FURTHER DEVELOPMENT OF HOSPICE CARE IN ISRAEL

We believe that at least in part because of the successful experience of the Tel Hashomer Hospice, there has been a rapid and impressive development of hospice care in many regions in Israel. In 1982 there were no hospices in this country. In 1983 there were two hospices. Today there are 20 hospices situated throughout the country, from the Lebanese border in the north to the Negev in the south. There are now four hospices per million population, providing 1.1 inpatient hospice beds per 100,000 population. In 1992, 6560 cancer patients died in Israel, of whom 1126 (17%) were directly cared for by a hospice. Furthermore, during the period from 1984 to 1992, Israel saw the most rapid rise of any country in the world in the consumption of morphine, which is widely regarded as an index of pain control services.

In 1993 the Israel Palliative Care Association (IPA) was established, and in 1995 the IPA was admitted to the European Association of Palliative Care as a collective member. The IPA publishes a newsletter, *Tmicha* (Support) three times a year and sponsors lectures and workshops. In 1996 we inaugurated a 120-hour course in palliative care for physicians, under the auspices of the Department of Family Medicine of Ben Gurion University of the Negev.

## HOSPICE AND JEWISH VALUES

It is interesting how a model of care with deep and ancient Christian roots has adapted itself so successfully to the religious and cultural traditions of the Jewish state. In fact, there is no fundamental contradiction between the approach of hospice and the approach of *halakha* (the Jewish legal system) to the dying patient. Both approaches emphasize:

- The holiness of life;
- The unacceptability of shortening a person's life; and
- The intensive care of the dying patient

Nonetheless, *halakha* does present some theoretical objections to the hospice approach. For example, *halakha* does not allow any defection from the ethical obligation to preserve life at all costs. Furthermore, *halakha* ordinarily would not countenance the withholding of parenteral fluid and nutrition. Our own research in this area would suggest, however, that providing parenteral nutrition and hydration does not extend the lifespan and may, in fact, be a source of additional discomfort for the dying patient. Therefore, the *halakhic* position and our own practice prove to be reconcilable on the basis of deeper medical understanding. Thus, although it is sometimes challenging to match the requirements of Jewish religious law to the approach of palliative care, there is no fundamental contradiction between the two. When difficult questions have arisen in individual cases, we have sought rabbinical advice, according to the wishes of the patient.

It is useful to remember that the care of the dying in the medieval Jewish *hekdesh* was similar to that in Christian hospices of the same period. The tradition of caring for the dying persist in both religious cultures as part of our common heritage. And it is precisely the absence of any fundamental contradiction between *halakha* and hospice that has enabled the rapid and thorough integration of palliative care within the Israeli medical system.

## CONCLUSION

During its 13 years of activity to this point, Tel Hashomer Hospice has not only provided good and appropriate treatment to patients in the terminal stages of cancer, but has also strengthened the awareness of their particular needs—among the Israeli medical community and Israeli society at large. By its successful example, the Tel Hashomer Hospice has stimulated the establishment of additional hospices throughout Israel. Ours was truly an international effort, for since our very first days we enjoyed the friendship, dvice, and support of colleagues abroad, most notably our English friends and especially those from St. Christopher's Hospice.

# REFERENCES

Olsen, S. L. (1988). Hospice administration: A life cycle model. *American Journal of Hospice Care, 5*, 40–47.

Waller, A., & Caroline N. (Eds.) (1996). *Handbook of palliative care in Cancer.* Boston: Butterworth-Heinemann.

# 23

# The Hospice Experience in Jordan: Al-Malath Foundation for Humanistic Care

Rana Hammad, MD*

The Hashemiat Kingdom of Jordan is an Arab country with a land area of 91,860 square miles. Jordan is bordered by Syria to the north, Iraq to the east, Saudi Arabia to the south, and Israel and the Palestinian Territories to the west. In 1993, the population of Jordan was estimated at 4,152,000, according to the Department of Statistics. This figure represents a 95% increase over the 1979 official census. The rise in population stems from the continuing high total fertility rate, decreasing mortality rate, and increasing overall life expectancy. The population increase has also been boosted by migration, particularly during the Gulf Crisis.

---

* To my mother . . . Your soul is always guiding me; to my husband and children . . . Your joyful spirit, support and patience made life easier; to my colleagues . . . Your support and cooperation made this dream a reality; and to Malath volunteers, families and supporters . . . You helped in enhancing the quality of life of many suffering people.

Amman, the capital, is inhabited by 1,231,000 people. The vast majority of the population are Sunni Muslims. Christians comprise about 4% of the total population. On the whole, Muslims and Christians coexist amicably, sharing the same culture.

The health care situation in Jordan has some imbalances that the government is attempting to overcome. In 1994, there was one physician for every 625 people, but only one nurse for every 1,087 (Ministry of Health, 1994). The same trend can be seen in professional standards. The quality of Jordan's surgeons is high, but nursing personnel are in short supply. Another problem is that hospitals are found only in the major urban centers. The government has made improvement of rural primary health care a high priority by establishing health centers capable of offering a wide range of services.

Health insurance plans available in Jordan do not comprehensively cover all the population. Some people in Jordan are not covered by any kind of health insurance, so they have to find their own funds to pay for health care. It is a different situation with cancer care, however. The governmental cancer health insurance programs covers 90% of the costs for health care for any person with cancer. Because the focus is on the curative approach, extensive use of technology, and long hospitalization periods, cancer care in Jordan is very costly to the government.

## TOWARD PALLIATIVE CARE

Although medical efforts are directed toward curing or controlling cancer, these goals sometimes cannot be achieved. It is at this point that the intervention must shift to palliation.

In Jordan and other Arab countries, there were no institutions or programs for the care of the terminally ill until 1992. At that time, a group of interested Jordanian professionals started meeting to explore the needs of the terminally ill and their families, and to consider the feasibility of a hospice home care program. All members of this group were knowledgeable about the needs and available services for terminally ill people in Jordan. They were also informed regarding the function and value of hospice care programs in other nations.

The concepts of palliative care and hospice services were not introduced formally in Jordan, nor were they included in medical and nursing curriculums. However, most of the health care professionals who had their postgraduate education in the United States or the Untied Kingdom had become familiar with these concepts. Returning to Jordan full of new ideas and an enthusiastic spirit, each of these professionals had a dream in mind. All that they needed was the opportunity to team up and cooperate, to establish a vehicle through which they could start a hospice care program in Jordan.

# PROGRAM JUSTIFICATION

The need for such a comprehensive service was also recognized by a group of concerned people in the community—health care professionals, religious leaders, social workers, and businessmen. These people met regularly and established a steering committee whose main task was to conceptualize the establishment of a hospice and palliative care service in Amman. It was a great help to have an American hospice nurse living in Jordan in 1992: Mrs. JoAnn Harisson, the wife of the American ambassador. She was an active participant in the steering committee, as was Mrs. Joan Marry Majali, a British nurse and the wife of the Jordanian Prime Minister.

The steering committee realized that the hospice vision would not be actualized unless it was shared with more and more people who could carry the message to others with enthusiasm. The first to respond to the idea of establishing a palliative care program for terminally ill patients were health care professionals who felt dissatisfied with the care provided within the current health care system. Many of these doctors and nurses had also had painful personal experience with relatives and friends who were dying from cancer. There was tension between the feeling of dissatisfaction with the health care provided to terminally ill patients and the new knowledge and skill that had become available. This tension contributed to the desire for change.

Interviews were conducted with religious leaders and health care professionals at the three largest hospitals in Amman: Jordan University Hospital, King Hussein Medical Center, and Al-Basheer Hospital. Additional interviews were conducted at an institute for specialized nursing studies, and an assessment of home-based nursing care for the terminally ill was conducted by a consultant from the International Hospice Institute.

It was concluded that there were no programs in Jordan that addressed the palliative care needs of the terminally ill or their families. A review of the literature revealed a study that had been conducted by two of the Mcmillan Nurses who were invited to Jordan to help in assessing cancer care and to help implement plans to develop care of the dying. The Mcmillan report of 1986 was thoughtfully and sensitively executed, raising many issues that required attention. Several references were made to standards of oncology nurses being "extremely high," but there was confusion between oncology and palliative care (Brown & Kay, 1986). The issue of *autonomy* was emphasized as being vitally important to remove barriers to direct interaction and communication between the dying person, the nurse, and the family. The problem of *pain control* was underscored as the chief reason for readmission to the hospital. This problem was seen as closely related to the issue of *legal restriction* on the prescription of adequate analgesics. These limitations had made pain control impossible in many instances, causing great distress to patients, family members, and medical staff.

It was concluded from a 1992 feasibility study that cancer is the third leading cause of death in Jordan after cardiovascular disorders and accidents. In 1991, 2,316 patients were treated for cancer at Jordan University Hospital while 1,214 new cases were diagnosed that year (Ministry of Health 1988). The Nuclear Medicine Department of Al-Basheer Hospital treated 1,323 new cases in 1993, and 2,074 additional patients in the Chemotherapy Department (Al-Basheer Hospital, 1993). At present, there are no accurate comprehensive statistics available on the number and types of cancer cases in Jordan, but some of the available statistics indicate that the number of cancer cases is rising.

The establishment of The Amal Cancer Center in Jordan, with its mission to provide curative care for cancer patients, will create a need for palliative care for those who have no hope for a cure. Additionally, there will be a need for support services for the families and the health care professionals who care for them.

As in most Middle Eastern nations, the sick, the elderly, and the dying usually are cared for at home by their families. Some people in Jordan die in hospitals, but most patients who are considered incurable are sent home from the hospital a few days before death. With only 2.55% of all patients dying in hospitals in Jordan, we can conclude that most patients do die at home.

Jordanians have strong traditions of hospitality and mutual caring. Families, friends, and even neighbors willingly and continuously look after terminally ill patients. When you observe Jordanian families surrounding their patients, you understand that the hospice philosophy is spontaneous and indigenous within the culture. Providing this kind of care is regarded as honorable work in Jordan. In our effort to provide high quality and cost-effective care, we seek to combine the age-old traditions of caring families in our society with current knowledge and skills of trained professionals.

As already noted, the usual course of management for terminally ill cancer patients in Jordan is mainly curative in goals and technique. Patients are treated in acute care settings as needed. When discharged from the hospitals, the patients would have only their family members available to provide care. No home care-based agency was available, except a few private nursing agencies that were expensive and not covered by any kind of insurance. With the increasing incidence of cancer and the late diagnosis of many cases, the majority of patients were left untreated and discharged to die at home.

Changes in the social structure of the family in Jordan and the lack of professional support systems have reduced the care that is supposed to be given to the patients by their families at home. Eventually, the patients are hospitalized again to die in hospitals. A conflict situation develops, as hospitals sometimes refuse to admit patients again while families exert pressure for readmission. Many patients die on their way to the emergency room or at its entrance, with frightened families and helpless professionals bitterly blaming each other.

Even if patients are admitted to hospitals, the situation is not necessarily any better. Patients with incurable illnesses often are considered to be medical failures, so there is a tendency to avoid them. Other patients are treated aggressively by physicians because they are urged to do so by the family. These patients are thereby subjected to technologically advanced but fruitless treatment methods as one alternative after another fails. Health care professionals are not well-trained to meet the needs of dying patients and their families. All hospital systems are acute care-oriented, so the care of these patients and their families was either fitted into the hospital's care orientation or—which is more likely—these cases were avoided.

During my postgraduate training in a pediatric oncology unit in one of the largest educational hospices in Jordan, I noticed that terminally ill cancer children did not receive good care. In my effort to learn the reason, I spared three full days for continuous observation. I sat at the entrance of the pediatric ward from 7 A.M. until 3 P.M. for 3 days. I counted the number of times a staff nurse entered the room of a terminally ill child as compared to the room of an acutely ill child.

To my surprise, I found that the staff nurse, on average, entered an acutely ill child's room about 20 times per shift—but the terminally ill child's room only five times per shift. These observations led to a new question: "Why?" The majority of nurses answered: "There is nothing we can do for them." Other nurses bravely admitted that they were avoiding terminally ill children. One of them said, "I don't want to be emotionally involved with them, because I will not be able to cope with my grief when they die . . . I should protect myself from stressors and burnout."

Jordan is a socially oriented country in which the people are capable of relating and interacting easily with each other. We have a deep religious and cultural belief that death is an inevitable fate and that every soul will taste it. Nevertheless, we are not accustomed to speak openly about our inner fears, especially in the area of dying and death. It is a cultural habit among Jordanians to encourage sick people and give them hope for cure. You will always hear visitors say upon entering the patient's room, "Oh, you look better today, and, of course, you will be much better tomorrow." When the visitors leave the room they immediately start crying, knowing the patient is dying.

## THE HOSPICE VISION

After a survey of the existing situation in Jordan and assessment of the need for a hospice service, the steering committee was able to envision a hospice program and design an initial plan of work. The hospice vision included a feeling of compassion for dying persons and their families, as well as demonstrable evidence that terminally ill patients can be made more comfortable at less expense. The commitee also realized that it was the right time to start the service. It was a priority to help others realize the obstacles to improved care of the dying. Our efforts were, therefore, aimed at spreading the message that it is a modern superstition to avoid acknowledgement of death, to treat it as though it were something unnatural, shameful, or wrong. It is mistaken as well to be extra-heroic or extra-passive with the claim that there is nothing more to be done. It is time to root out the fears and misconceptions that lie behind this distorted view. We must begin to honor the labor of those who are about to complete their journey. This is our mission.

We concluded that there is talent, interest, and some individually developed expertise in Jordan concerning terminal and palliative care which needed to be coordinated and guided to help in developing palliative care services and a national awareness of its importance.

## PALLIATIVE CARE AND THE COMMUNITY

It was very helpful to discuss the hospice idea with health care professionals and colleagues. As these health care providers are also actual or potential health care consumers, their observations from both personal and professional perspectives were useful and significant. The health care providers reported great discomfort and dissatisfaction with the way in which the terminally ill and their families are treated. They reported an absence of support for the families, the practice of keeping information away from patients, unrealistic fears of contagion, and the absence of religious support. In addition, they recognized that patients and families often have anxiety about death—and that many religious leaders seem to be more concerned with instructing people about the rules and regulations they should follow than with offering guidance and comfort.

Health care professionals and the community appear to be very supportive of the hospice idea. It is felt that these services will help people better understand how to take care of their terminally ill family members, and to accept their condition. It will also enable those who are terminally ill to die peacefully at home surrounded by their families, instead of in institutional isolation.

The health care professionals reported feeling lost in trying to meet the needs of their patients while at the same time trying to meet their own needs. Many also mentioned difficulties in dealing with their own grief. Communication issues were a major source of concern for the nurses, because great efforts are made to keep patients unaware of the nature of their terminal condition, especially when it is cancer. Nurses are caught between the patients' requests to know what is happening to them, and the family's wish to protect patients from knowing the truth.

My friends and family members were strongly supportive when I discussed the idea of a hospice program—and why not, when each person can see him- or herself as a potential incurable case one day! Each person is vulnerable to the fear of having cancer, and the fear of lingering illness, suffering, and pain. Having become involved voluntarily in establishing the hospice program immediately after my mother's death, I was not quite sure about my own ability to deal with dying people. I was afraid that this desire might prove to be a short-term impulse that would quickly fade. I remember the courage and determination I gained after talking with my father, who was still grieving my mother when he said to me: "We were blessed, and so was she when she died having us surrounding her with all the love and care possible. . . . You should work hard to help other families capture the best of their moments together the way we did. . . ."

## THE BEGINNING

Six months of continuous work, data gathering, and networking passed before the proposed program was articulated. The second stage was the responsibility of the professional working group, which steamed up from the steering committee. During the next few months, more information was obtained, while meetings and the recruitment of additional people continued. Key health care people and community activists were included, and each had a role to play in the establishment of the hospice service.

Our efforts were crowned in February, 1993, by the formal registration of the project as a nongovernmental society under the umbrella of the General Union for Voluntary Societies (GUVS) at the Ministry of Social Development. The hospice concept was thereby introduced in Jordan. The nonprofit volunteer organization took the name "The Malath Foundation for Humanistic Care." *Malath* is an Arabic word that means "the last shelter" or "choice." This word is used to describe the care given to people who have nowhere else to go.

The Foundation has an elected board of directors which is responsible for fundraising and major policy decisions. The day-to-day operations are overseen by the professional working group, which is supported by four committees made up of volunteers. These committees are: Education and Training, Patient Management, Fund Raising and Marketing, and Spiritual and Bereavement. The commitees meet on a regular basis and report back to the professional group.

Volunteers usually are not involved in direct patient care because family members and relatives assume this responsibility under our supervision. Occasionally, we face a problem in coordinating the huge number of relatives who volunteer to help. The volunteers do help in some cases, though, with shopping, cooking, and babysitting, under the supervision of the attending nurse. Professional nurses volunteer to provide direct patient care. Malath volunteers primarily are professionals who have full-time jobs. Few volunteers can give more than four hours of service per week. Consequently, it is almost impossible to enroll the volunteers in any formal training program. Instead, we arrange for special informal educational activities.

## RESISTANCE

Since it was only a dream at first, our hospice care project did not always seem to be an excellent idea to everybody. A few health care professionals were antagonistic. This response occurred mostly among some traditional doctors and nurses who were not comfortable with innovations that were modifying or replacing their familiar practices. These opponents could not imagine how health care could be provided if control was given to the patients and their relatives.

Many others were not antagonistic, but, rather, skeptical. Their arguments focused on how difficult it would be to actualize the hospice vision. It was their view that even the most strenuous efforts to introduce hospice care would fail because there was no suitable comprehensive health system in which the new approach could be integrated. We could not accept this obstacle as insurmountable, however, because we knew at the beginning that there was no existing system to support us—we would have to work hard to create that system!

Day by day, the hospice experience expanded. With each new case it was demonstrated that palliative care is the most humane alternative in the care of terminally ill patients. The skeptics started to realize that it is much harder to deal with dying and death when one cannot do anything that is helpful. They discovered through hospice that there were ways to help patients, families, and themselves. Only then did they come to appreciate the comfort and dignity that is provided by the palliative care approach and that every human deserves. Gradually but surely, some of those who were skeptical at the beginning started to join the project as volunteers and supporters.

Resistance is natural within a process of change, and should be handled carefully. The resistance we encountered was expected because we were introducing unfamiliar concepts. While accurately evaluating the nature and possible causes of this resistance, we were very careful neither to underestimate it or deal with it on a personal level.

## CHALLENGES

The Foundation faces several challenges in attempting to achieve its goals. Funding strategies needed to be developed to make this program successful and accessible to all those in need of its services. The expenses associated with starting the program were covered by a grant allocated to Al-Malath by The United States Agency for International Development (USAID) and GUVS. This grant was utilized to invite a consult to assist in conducting workshops, in training members of the Foundation abroad, and in purchasing equipment for patient care and a car for team transportation.

Since this startup support, we faced many financial challenges. The hardest was to attract the needed money to rent and furnish an office, because at that time only a few people knew about us. We had to adopt a different strategy in fundraising, that of approaching only those people known to be supportive of pioneer projects. After a full year of operating the hospice from our houses, we were finally able to rent and furnish a three-room office. Since then, we have accelerated our services. This activity has included recruiting and training staff as well as admitting more and more patients.

The next financial challenge then emerged: how to sustain our work. It was somewhat easier to obtain funding by this time, however, because more people had heard about our services, especially after continuous media coverage. Furthermore, everybody could see that the money donated was being used for good patient care and for useful educational services.

Up to this point in time, the Foundation has not received any kind of payment, neither for patient care nor for lectures and workshops. All our money is obtained from individual and family donations and fundraising activities. However, for the hospice to remain a viable medical, community, and national resource, it will be necessary to have services paid for in the future through a sliding scale fee based on family income. If the social worker determines that a family is below the poverty level, then a small payment will be agreed upon to give a sense of value and contribution to the service. It is the Foundation's belief that no one should be denied care because of financial need. To maintain this mission, we will develop and implement additional fund raising strategies, as well as approaching governmental and private institutions.

Another challenge we face is the public's limited awareness of the hospice concept and the availability of palliative care services. Although there is a need for additional palliative care programs in Jordan, we still need to encourage people to take advantage of the existing program. People often are reluctant to contact us because they do not know exactly what we can do. We are faced with almost the same comment from both doctors and family members: "What can you do for your patients since they are dying?" It takes only two or three visits from Al-Malath team members to demonstrate what we do and how it makes a difference in the quality of care.

Usually, patients are referred to us in the later stages of their illness. The average stay for our patients is 28 days, so we still need to encourage physicians to refer their patients earlier in order to meet their needs more fully. We expected community physicians to start referring their patients to the hospice program after we had cared for several. We still need to go back to them, however, and ask them to refer more patients to us. The limited flow of patients is probably related to the fact that we have focused more on educating nurses than on physicians. The majority of our educational activities targeted nurses and the general public. As a result, nurses, families, and friends are more cooperative with us than are physicians, and are the major sources of patient referrals. If we could go back in time and replan our educational programs, we definitely would have given equal emphasis from the start to educating both nurses and doctors, as well as the community.

The involvement of clergy in palliative care programs in our region is a new concept that must be understood, developed, and implemented. To meet this challenge, the Foundation has recruited several clergymen to its spiritual committee. These clergymen have been educated on palliative care and the goals of the Foundation's program. They have worked together in discussing and defining their role in palliative care and the way to provide spiritual support to the terminally ill and their families.

Our initial plan was to form an active group of clergy who would provide spiritual support to terminally ill patients and their families. Surprisingly, however, families and patients almost never have asked for spiritual support, and are likely to refuse it when offered. Instead, families prefer to support their patient themselves. This finding led us to have our nurses mentored by clergymen on how to support their patients and families. The spiritual aspect of care now is provided by nurses. Clergy are called in when and if the family expresses a wish for their involvement.

Pain control continues to be a major challenge. Most physicians and nurses have not been trained in pain control. There is a great fear that patients might become addicted to pain control drugs. The other issue related to pain control is the availability of drugs. In Jordan, the drug and narcotic law is very rigid. It allows for a prescription that is adequate for only three days of pain control. Furthermore, the prescription can be dispensed only by a limited number of pharmacies in the public sector. Making the situation even more difficult is the fact that the the only forms of morphine available in Jordan are injections and the sustained-release MST 30 or 60 mg tablets.

These restrictions cause great frustration for patients and their families, as well as for their physicians, who feel helpless in trying to relieve their patient's suffering. In many cases, physicians have to admit patients to hospitals to control their pain more effectively.

It was a priority of ours to work closely with the Minister of Health in reviewing the narcotics control law, as well as developing and implementing regulations that would decentralize dispensing of narcotics, and insure longer prescription periods. We had expected to work on this issue for several years. Fortunately, however, the Ministry of Health understood the situation and recognized that many people supported the palliative care concept. The regulations have now been changed to increase the number of tablets per prescription and decentralize morphine dispensing. These changes have made it easier for physicians to control their patient's pain, and also save a lot of time and effort for families.

Although the liberalization of pain-control medications was a great and unexpected achievement, our largest achievement was beyond our plans. In our effort to create a system in which palliative care could be established in Jordan, we urged the Ministry of Health to establish a national task force representing all health sectors, with its main task to be the development of a comprehensive national cancer policy. Again, with the understanding and cooperation of the Ministry of Health, a national committee was formed for this purpose. It is our hope that the end result of this work will be a new system guided by a comprehensive national cancer control policy—with palliative care programs included.

Our efforts were boosted by the cooperation of the World Health Organization (WHO) and the Eastern Mediterranean Region Office (EMR). A regional training course on cancer pain and palliative care was prepared by the pain unit of the WHO in Geneva and EMR. As the only hospice program in the region, the Al-Malath Foundation had a major role in preparing and implementing the training course, held in June, 1995. The outcomes of the course were beyond all expectations. It is stimulating all other countries in the region to develop their own national cancer control policies, including palliative care programs. This successful and highly stimulating conference was not only our best achievement so far, but it has given rise to a new horizon that promises future plans and achievements.

## FUTURE PLANS

Our hospice program has targeted adult cancer patients almost exclusively. We need to develop new programs for children and for patients with other forms of chronic disease as well. We realize that more effort is needed in this area. As Peter Kay has observed:

> The concept of applying the principles of palliative medicine to neurological and rheumatological diseases implies huge changes in thinking about priorities in medicine and resource allocation. It also requires adoption of new attitudes by all the caring professions, especially those of medicine and nursing. A change in professional priority from cure to care, from intervention to prevention and rehabilitation, becomes not only desirable but economic. If this is to be achieved, the hospice will have much to do in leading the way (Kaye, 1992).

Our future plans also include the development of trained palliative care teams working in all the hospitals where cancer patients are treated. Other teams will be developed to enhance community outreach by serving patients outside the capital, Amman. We are also planning to establish an inpatient unit that will serve the living as well as the dying. It will function as a community resource for advising other health professionals on palliative care issues. It will make valuable services, such as those of the pain and physiotherapy clinic and the education and research center, available to all patients. The inpatient unit will serve as a backup for the home care program with its responsibilties for diagnostic workup, assessment, evaluation, monitoring, and the management of pain and other symptoms. The inpatient program will come into play when the scope of the patient's medical problem does not allow for care in the home setting. It will also coordinate with home care teams in providing a comprehensive service package to patients and their families.

When fully established and operational, the Foundation will foster clinical care experiences for both nursing and medical students, as well as the organization of workshops in palliative care and bereavement.

## SOME THOUGHTS FOR FUTURE HOSPICE PIONEERS

As founders of a pioneering hospice program in the Middle East, we realize that our project faces many challenges at both the local and national levels. The success of our experience so far has been due in large part to creative and committed professionals and volunteers and to the sharing of information and resources. In additional, a wide variety of collaborative efforts have promoted the hospice concept and advocated for its inclusion as a legitimate and recognized health care alternative for terminally ill people and their families. These same activities will continue to be essential as the hospice movement matures, stabilizes, and grows to meet new demands.

It was difficult to develop a culturally acceptable model of care because there were no similar models in the region to draw upon. The experience was exactly like that of climbing a mountain. Whenever you reach a top, a new top appears at the horizon. Occasionally, you will feel that you are not achieving anything. If you pause a little and look back, though, you will appreciate the distance you have walked.

If you are considering starting a palliative care program, remember that determination and networking are the keys. Knowing that the time is right to start a program in your country and recognizing that it is much needed does not mean that you have to force yourself to rush. We always need to go ahead-slowly and steadily in such circumstances. If we seek to induce a long-lasting change, we must work on changing attitudes and focus on re-education, rather than allowing ourselves to become over-hurried in the hope of achieving a quick turnaround.

# REFERENCES

Al-Basheer Hospital. Nuclear Medicine Department. (1993). *The annual report*. Amman, Jordan: Author.

Brown, A., & Kay, J. (1986). *The continuing care of the patient with advanced cancer*. Unpublished manuscript.

Jordan Ministry of Health. (1994). *The annual statistical report*. Amman, Jordan: Author.

Jordan Ministry of Health. (1988). *The annual statistical report*. Amman, Jordan: Author.

Kaye, P. (1992). *A to Z of hospice and palliative medicine*. London: Cynthia Spencer House.

# 24

# Palliative Care for the Terminally Ill in Saudi Arabia

Alan J. Gray, MD, A. Ezzart, MD, and A. Boyar, MD

## HEALTH CARE IN SAUDI ARABIA

Saudi Arabia has a population of approximately 17 million people, of whom 13 million are Saudi nationals and 4 million expatriates. It resembles other developing nations in its youthfulness (half the population is under the age of 16) and relatively large family size (seven children on the average). The growth rate is the highest in the world: a 3.5% annual increase. Saudi Arabia has undergone many dramatic technological changes. The oil-based economy transformed Saudi Arabia from a mainly nomadic to a predominantly urban society with a sophisticated infrastructure of industry, transportation, communications, education, and health systems—and all of this within a space of 20–30 years.

In previous times, the Saudi population suffered the infectious diseases common in underdeveloped countries, including tuberculosis and malaria. These conditions have now been very successfully controlled by innovative vaccination and public health programs, and no longer pose a major threat. The average life expectancy has risen markedly as a result of these improvements. It is estimated that men and women in the Middle East as a whole have an average life expectancy of only 62 years, compared with the West where life expectancy is 75 years or more. However, Saudi Arabia has already reached an average life expectancy of 70 years. This increase is most likely associated with the rapid improvements in nutrition, sanitation, housing, and maternity care, along with vaccination programs.

Along with most other countries, the population of Saudi Arabia is undergoing an epidemiological transition in which the morbidity and mortality patterns are changing from those associated with infectious diseases and nutritional deficiencies to what some have called "the age of degenerative and man-made diseases" such as cancer, heart, and cerebrovascular disease. It can be predicted with reasonable assurance that this, combined with the prolongation of life expectancy, will lead to an absolute increase in the number of cases of cancer occurring in the Kingdom. An increasing proportion of these cases will occur in older people. In Kuwait and Bahrain, where population-based statistics are available, cancer is already the most common cause of death. Cancer does, of course, occur at any age, and Saudi Arabia with its large proportion of young people has a significant problem with cancer in children. Children comprise 13% of the cancer patients seen at King Faisal Specialist Hospital and Research Centre (KFSH & RC), a larger proportion of the total cancer cases than are seen in similar referral centers in the West.

Saudi Arabia has yet to develop the level of personal sophistication in health matters or the depth of primary health care care delivery to make earlier diagnoses and, therefore, begin treatment sooner. Seventy percent of the adult cancer patients seen at KFSH & RC (the major tertiary health care center for the Kingdom) present with advanced stage cancer (stages 3 or 4). Nevertheless, all these patients are accepted with the prospect of successful treatment by surgery, chemotherapy, or radiotherapy. For an unselected population of patients in a Western country, the number would be approximately 30% at stage 3 or 4.

In 1989, a group of nurses at KFSH & RC met informally and considered the need for a Home Health Care Program for seriously ill patients in the Riyadh area, a city of over 3 million people and the capital city of Saudi Arabia. Many of these countries, such as the Yemen and the Sudan, have underdeveloped medical care systems. These patients arrive with the expectation that their advanced cancer will somehow be cured, and their symptoms relieved. Many of these patients, however, have cancer which cannot be treated successfully. Previous, these patients were sent home without relief or recommendations for supportive care from their local health centers.

Furthermore, many referring physicians did not recognize the need to look after dying cancer patients in their own region. This attitude may have been related to their lack of confidence, skills, and local resources. Patients who do receive ongoing treatment at KFSH & RC, and whose disease is relapsing, rely on this hospital for their total care. They often come to the emergency service for symptom management. Patients fear discharge from this hospital, as it could mean abrupt cessation of the high quality medical care they have been receiving.

## THE BEGINNINGS OF PALLIATIVE CARE IN SAUDI ARABIA

In 1989, a group of nurses at KFSH & RC met informally and considered the need for a home health care program for seriously ill patients in the Riyadh area. A proposal was formulated and accepted by the hospital administration, which established a task force to design and implement a pilot study to assess its feasibility. A questionnaire was sent to patients, families, nurses, and physicians to survey their attitudes toward such a concept. The results of the survey were encouraging. There was concern about the language barrier, however, and the possible negative responses from Saudi families to the idea of non-Saudi females entering their homes to care for family members.

A pilot study was approved in February, 1990 and implemented over a four-month period. This study included 12 patients in the terminal stages of cancer. Nine of these patients died at home, and three in other hospitals. The results indicated that patients and families benefited from the nursing care and psychosocial support. Patients and their families were very receptive to the advice and care given by the nurses and welcomed them to their homes with friendship, respect, and hospitality. The study also demonstrated that such a program reduced the need for hospital admissions and clinic and emergency visits, thereby contributing to the judicious use of hospital resources and staff time. The program was also found to have enhanced the Hospital's public relations.

Approval was soon given to establish a home health care program under the supervision of a committee to oversee its ongoing planning and implementation. The program was under the direction of a medical director and a head nurse. There were also four staff nurses, four translators/drivers who are Saudi males, a social worker, a secretary, and a messenger. Nursing requirements included experience in community nursing, a working knowledge of Arabic, and a sensitive, caring, and nonjudgmental approach to patient care in a different cultural setting. The service was to include the chronically ill as well as the terminally ill. This Home Health Care Service was the first of its kind in the Kingdom.

Later in the same year, Dr. Derek Doyle, medical director of Edinburgh's St. Columba's Hospice, was invited to visit and advise on the service. His report made specific recommendations on the further development of the Home Health Care Service, the appointment of a specialist in palliative care, and the development of a consultative team for inpatients, together with an inpatient unit. He also identified the need for an educational program to create awareness and improve skills generally. Doyle recommended the preparation of guidelines on ethical issues as they relate to information for patients and their families, as well as the need to educate expatriate staff on Islamic and Arabic culture as related to dying, death, and grief.

# THE PALLIATIVE CARE PROGRAM TODAY AND ITS CHALLENGES

At present, a multidisciplinary team provides total care for the patient and support for the patient as a unit. This team includes the part-time services of a consultant oncologist with a background in palliative care, and a full-time physician working as a palliative care consultant, together with six professional nurses, five translators/drivers, and a social worker. The team consults with professionals in other health disciplines to provide the most appropriate care. The service runs 24 hours, 7 days a week.

So far, approximately 900 patients have been referred to the program, but this includes a number of people with chronic as well as terminal illness. Palliative care for a terminal illness makes up 75% of the work load. At any one time there are between 80–100 patients in the community, of whom 40 to 50 have a terminal illness. Four inpatient beds are provided in the hospital for symptom control. About 25 patients per month are admitted to these beds, and approximately 60% of these patients are able to be discharged home again.

Five major problems exist currently:

## 1. Primary, Secondary, and Care Services

The Kingdom lacks a well-developed system of primary health care services with a network of family doctors and community nurses who know and understand the patients and their families. Intead, primary health care is provided through a system of polyclinics. These clinics provide effective vaccination programs for children, as well as many other services, but do not appear to be involved in continuing care for chronic illness. Their care seems more concentrated on acute episodes of illness.

The Kingdom is served by a system of 174 public hospitals, and has numerous private clinics. For a patient with either a chronic or a terminal illness, continuing care even in the community tends to be provided by the hospital service. The aim should be to drive this type of care into the primary health system.

## 2. Cure Versus Palliation

The emphasis is on "curative treatment" for cancer patients in Saudi Arabia. It is not always recognized by clinicians that palliative care may be appropriate for some patients. This interface between curative cancer treatment and palliative care will improve only when clinicians see the benefits of a palliative care program and what it can achieve for their patients.

The problem is compounded by the relationship between the doctor and the patient here, which differs from that of Western countries. In the West, health care systems are based on the individual. Patients are regarded as autonomous agents capable of receiving information and making decisions about their own future. The predominant principle in Saudi Arabia, however, is one of "beneficience." The patient is viewed as one member of the larger family, and it is the family that is responsible for the patient.

The consent of the patient to treatment usually takes the form of a substitute consent by the family. The purpose of this practice is to avoid disturbing the patient emotionally. The family believes it is protecting the patient from harm and ensuring that treatment is carried out in an ethical manner.

It is assumed that an ill patient will not adapt to the situation of terminal illness. According to this way of thinking, awareness of terminal illness results in a loss of hope which may lead to an earlier death. This concept of denying patients information on their terminal illness is shared by many other nations, of course. This policify of beneficience also relies on the perception of health professionals as authority figures who can be trusted to do what is best for the patient. We need to develop to a stage where patients and families have greater trust that the health program will relieve their symptoms, whatever the stage of the cancer, and that "no cure" will not be the same as "no care."

The introduction of modern medical technology is also changing the relationship between patient and doctor. Such technology has a "cost" to the patients in terms of toxicity, as well as major benefits. Increasingly, physicians dealing with cancer and other major illnesses here insist that the patient be fully informed and able to give consent before starting a treatment that will have side effects. Already, many patients in this country are well-informed about their illness and have some idea of their prognosis. This trend will increase steadily as more young Saudi doctors return from training in Europe and North America with Western ideas of communicating with patients.

## 3. Pain Relief

There is a general lack of knowledge of how and when to use morphine effectively. Moreover, morphine is simply not available in most of the Kingdom. Even Demerol is restricted, and there is a general reluctance to use analgesics of any kind. There is an unreasonable fear of morphine addiction among patients and their families in the Kingdom.

At KFSH & RC, however, we use morphine in a manner very similar to the way it is used in the West. We have long-acting morphine tablets available and use subcutaneous morphine infusions, at home or in hospital. However, we are one of only a handful of hospitals in the Kingdom that can use morphine for outpatients. There is an urgent need to disseminate the knowledge and technology of pain relief more widely. Addictive drugs of any kind are prohibited by Islam. This ban applies particularly to alcohol and narcotics, but in 1926 King Abdulasiz Ibn Saud also prohibited cigarette smoking, in all its forms, as not Islamic. Unfortunately, this particular ban has since elapsed.

These prohibitions have led to a natural reluctance by patients to take and for doctors to prescribe morphine. This resistance is usually overcome by continuous monitoring of patients by the home health care nurses, which results in better communication. Information pamphlets in Arabic are also helpful. Nevertheless, there are still patients who refuse to take morphine under any circumstances, despite their intense pain, and many doctors who refuse to prescribe morphine.

## 4. Cultural Aspects

Foreign health professionals are constantly impressed by the strength of family life in the Kingdom. The family unit is the structural foundation of Saudi society, and it appears that patients here cope better with a terminal illness at home than happens elsewhere. This advantage is probably the result of the close family involvement and strong Islamic faith which allows them to accept death as an expression of God's will. It is a religious duty to provide for parents in case of need, to help make their lives as comfortable as possible. Furthermore, modern medicine is a recent development, and older people are accustomed to enduring severe physical hardship.

At first, it was uncertain that foreign health professionals would be accepted into Saudi homes to care for chronically or terminally ill patients. Saudi homes are intensely private and protected. This concern proved unfounded. Hospitality is a very important part of Saudi culture, and nurses and doctors are welcomed and respected. Much of this success is due to the use of Saudi men as drivers and translators. These people provide a 24-hour service, look after the security of the nurses, act as social workers in assessing the needs of the family, and serve as the link between the patient and family, the nurse, and the doctor. The translators/ drivers are a remarkably dedicated and effective group of men who participate fully in the work of the team.

Nevertheless, it is extremely important to understand and respect the customs in the Kingdom. Hospitality is valued as one of the main elements in social life. It helps eradicate that social isolation which is not acceptable within Islam. It is important to notify the family of an intentioned visit. The women in the house must be given time to put on their veils or to retire to a part of the house where visitors will not enter. This practice can cause problems if the primary caregiver is a woman who retires to another part of the house when the nurse visits. The unavailability of the primary caregiver severely limits communication in attempting to assess the status of the patient. It is unusual to receive permission to visit unless there is a male member of the family present.

There are other important rules to observe. One must never interrupt people who are in prayer. Footwear must be left at the door. Nearly always the visitor is offered a drink, usually with food. It is impolite to refuse. Refreshment often provides an excellent opportunity to talk to the family about the patient's illness and explore their knowledge and fears.

During Ramadan, the family will be fasting during the day. Visiting can be difficult, because the family often is awake long into the night and spends much of the day sleeping. Even seriously ill patients often insist on fasting during Ramadan. They may also refuse medications during this period. Patients who are obviously dying may want to travel to Mecca for their last pilgraimage. Nearly always, this plan can be encouraged. An amazing number of patients whose general condition seems desperate make the pilgrimage to Mecca and return home before dying.

Older patients commonly sleep on a platform on the floor. Chairs are not normally a part of the furniture in a Saudi house. One become used to squatting or kneeling, as is the Saudi custom. Most women dislike showing their faces. Care and consideration are required at all stages of a physical examination. With gentle encouragement, cooperation is nearly always obtained.

The impression in this country is that a small input of medical and nursing care results in a magnified response by the extended family in the care of the patient. This can be very gratifying to the doctor and nurse. Although our home care program is a relatively small operation in terms of number of patients served, it instills new expectations about what good primary health care in the community can achieve. There is a "spin-off" to other members of the community through the network of the large extended families. The teaching involved in the care of one patient has the potential to influence larger numbers about their perception of the disease and what can be achieved. Ten or fifteen or even more people may observe and benefit from this education.

Unfortunately, there is still some confusion between palliative care and euthanasia—which is totally forbidden by Islam. Some interpret palliative care as equivalent to witholding treatment. For example, there is no forced feeding to an unconscious patient through a nasogastric tube. Many dying patients with cancer undergo surgery, chemotherapy, or radiotherapy, or may be sent overseas for treatment, all of which may not be appropriate. These futile interventions often occur because of the difficulties in discussing issues of prognosis, death, and dying.

Inappropriate surgery, the use of ineffective chemotherapy or radiotherapy, intensive care, and artificial respiration in a terminal illness are all examples of treatment from which the patient and relatives may be dissuaded through information and discussion. However, expatriate doctors may find it easier to respond to the patient's wishes rather than to discuss the issue in depth. Talking about life-and-death issues with the patient may make the physician feel too uncomfortable. Inappropriate medical treatments are therefore common, not only in this country, but also for many Saudi patients who go abroad, seeking further treatment in the medical market.

There is a need to educate the population that palliative care is the moral and ethical alternative to euthanasia: that it provides comfort and sustains hope. This society, quite rightly, sets great store by hope, and anything that diminishes hope is seen as diminishing the patient's life expectancy.

## 5. Work Force

The government employs 14,500 doctors, but only 12% are Saudi nationals. Nearly all of the 33,000 members of the nursing work force are expatriates. There is a constant turnover of expatriate staff. The commitment and continuing care required for good palliative care (and, indeed, the rest of medicine) is only likely to be fully realized when the majority of the work force are Saudi nationals.

Palliative care would make a good role model for teaching in Saudi medical and nursing schools. Traditional healers have an important supportive role in this society, and the potential exists for incorporating them into palliative care services.

## A CASE EXAMPLE

*Saeed, age 65, presented to KFSH & RC for treatment of an advanced gastric carcinoma. He gave a three-year history of abdominal pain that was treated initially with ranitidine. As his symptoms progressed, however, he turned to traditional Arabic medicine. Eventually, weight loss and fatigue led him to seek medical care elsewhere. Finally, he had an endoscopy, through which the gastric carcinoma was found, and he was sent to KFSH & RC for treatment.*

*Saeced came from a village 300 kilometers outside Riyadh. A surgical appointment was followed by laporotomy when widespread disease with nodal, and liver involvement was diagnosed. At this point, he was referred for palliative care and given medications to control his symptoms. Followup appointments were scheduled at weekly intervals. Saeed preferred to drive the 300 kilometers from his home for these appointments, rather than continue followup with his local medical service, although this option was offered to him.*

*After three weeks, he presented to the emergency room for acute bowel obstruction and was admitted to the hospital. His symptoms were controlled with a subcutaneous* infusion, but there was no relief of his bowel obstruction. His family became concerned about his need to be back home with them and to talk to a family elder about his will.

Saeed was the father of 20 children and the husband of three women. Despite the family's pressure, however, he was unwilling to transfer to a major hospital near his home. His family moved to a flat in Riyadh, and he was able to be discharged to their care under supervision by the Home Health Care Service until he died. His will had been made by then. Saeed's family appreciated the primary care provided by the Home Health Care Service. Prominent in the community, Saeed's family may be able to pass on the knowledge that effective services can be provided to terminally ill people to other families as their needs arise.

## CONCLUSION

The pilot program at KFSH & RC has proved that it is possible to provide palliative care of a similar standard to that in a Western country. It has also found that cultural values predominant in the Middle East actually enhance and promote this form of care. These cultural values include strong family bonds, the acceptance of matters of life and death as an expression of God's will, and the emphasis on hospitality.

The program continues to develop. At present, there is a proposal to involve other hospitals in the city, but the major need is for an educational program for health professionals nationwide. Saudi Arabia has the advantage of a government-funded and provided health service which can allow for rational planning on a national basis. The program at KFSH & RC has encountered the usual administrative difficulties, which have reaffirmed the value of the comprehensive mission statement that was developed by the original working group in 1991, as well as the need for regular reviews of the goals of the service.

# PART III
## Conclusion

# 25

# Hospice Care on the International Scene: Today and Tomorrow

## Robert Kastenbaum and Marilyn Wilson

Throughout this book, participants in the international hospice care movement have spoken for themselves in words and numbers. It is the purpose of the present chapter to offer a brief summary statement of what has been learned and an even briefer anticipation of future challenges and developments. Much that is useful and important in the preceding chapters is necessarily omitted here.

## BASIC FACTS

Several basic facts emerge from the information shared by the contributors to this book, including the hospice programs that responded to the questionnaire but were not individually profiled:

1. Hospice care programs have been established in countries and cultures that differ markedly from the United Kingdom, where the model services originated, and North America, where such services have been rapidly developed. It is already clear that palliative care concepts and techniques are not limited to any

one type of sociotechnological structure, any one level of economic development, or any one religious belief system.

2. All world cultures appear to have traditional strengths that can contribute to the success of a palliative care program. Particularly conspicuous are those strengths that are included under the rubric of "family values." Some characteristics of traditional culture may be resistant, at least initially, to hospice services, but the experiences reported in this book indicate that love and concern for dying members of the family and the community will take precedence and bring forth a warm and caring response.

3. The early phases of hospice development invariably encounter resistance from several quarters. Some medical practitioners, some governmental officials, and some powerful forces in the community often misinterpret and fear even the effort to discuss dying and terminal care openly. These resistances are not to be underestimated, but they often dissolve rapidly through educational efforts and, especially, when the profound benefits of hospice care become evident to everybody.

4. Pain relief remains a central, if not the most central, objective of palliative care. It is here that some of the most difficult problems of attitude change are encountered. Most hospice programs have had to work strenuously to persuade physicians and lawmakers that it is both essential and possible to relieve the suffering of terminally ill people without creating "drug addicts" or engaging in lethal interventions.

5. Local and national health care systems often lack the mandate, the structure, or the know-how to accommodate hospice programs. This frequently encountered situation has required hospice advocates to become astute and effective change agents in their country's overall health care system. Although this adds substantially to the challenge, it can also result in an even greater contribution to well-being: as health care systems orient themselves to the concepts of palliation, individual and family values, open discussion, and the caring team they also become more responsive in general to the needs of the public and the care providers.

6. Exceptional energy and persistence are required to develop and maintain a hospice care program. The character and dedication of a relatively few people are crucial in the early stages, where the hospice concept is not well known or accepted, and where there are numerous obstacles to overcome on every side. (The fact that the names of many individuals are mentioned in the foregoing chapters goes beyond courteous acknowledgement: the development of local hospice programs always requires the emergence of energetic, persistent, and innovative individuals.) Even when well established, however, hospice programs do not "run on automatic" and require continued passion, vigilance, flexibility, and dedication. In the most favorable circumstances, a larger and well-diversified set of people share this responsibility.

7. Financial support for hospice programs is generally a concern from the beginning, and remains a concern even when the benefits of palliative care have been well demonstrated. No hospice program has been able to say, "Now we are financially secure. Now we can provide all the necessary services to all those in need." The growing worldwide success of hospice programs in achieving its humanitarian goals has not guaranteed adequate continuing financial support; therefore, much effort must continue to be directed to fundraising efforts.

## FUTURE OF HOSPICE CARE THROUGHOUT THE WORLD

The brief and selective set of statements offered above apply to hospice care on the international scene today. Some of these statements also reveal present-day challenges that will have an effect on the future of hospice care (e.g., financial support). Now we focus on several other challenges and issues that hospice programs will need to deal with in the years immediately ahead.

1. Education of the general public, human service professionals, and governmental decisionmakers remains a significant challenge. Many people are still inadequately informed or misinformed about hospice care, even in countries where such programs have existed for 10 or 20 years. There is a tendency for fears and apprehensions to interfere at first with recognition of what hospice actually is and does. Educational efforts may need to be broader than clarification of palliative care *per se*. Hospice staff might well work in close collaboration (as they do in some areas) with death educators who attempt to deal with the entire spectrum of the human encounter with mortality. The "unthinkable" and the "unspeakable" must become acceptable subjects for open communication if hospice functions are to be conducted within a supportive sociocultural context. Decisionmakers must achieve emotional as well as cognitive learning experiences to realize the value of competent care for the terminally ill, and therefore not play politics with hospice programs. Professional education for physicians, nurses, and other care providers must not consider holistic palliative care as an optional frill, but as a core responsibility that must be understood by all who might be called upon to provide assistance to patients and families during the terminal process.

2. Sociotechnological change is creating a new and unprecedented context within which hospice care must operate. "Globalization" is one facet of this prevasive pattern of change. Once-distant parts of the world are becoming linked by satellites, e-mail, faxes, and other emerging technologies. Implications for hospice are likely to be varied, complex, and not entirely predictable. We have already seen that the St. Christopher's model of hospice care was discovered and adopted/adapted by care providers in many parts of the world. One may expect rapid dissemination of advances in knowledge and more immediate and versatile

modes for consultation by virtue of the new technologies. Globalization, however, also makes it possible for mistakes to take hold quickly, and even for abuse by individuals who might enter the system with personal agendas in mind.

Another facet of sociotechnological change is the combination of social destabilization and increasing diversity of population. Political and religious conflicts, often accompanied by violence, destruction of homes and farm lands, and "ethnic cleansing" have already generated a very large number of dispossessed people who seek shelter wherever it can be found. This process—which creates new responsibilities, stresses, and conflicts in the sheltering lands—might continue and even increase in the future. The enormous challenge of establishing hospice within a country as painfully destabilized as Colombia provides a vivid present example. Furthermore, people seeking economic opportunities in other countries have also entered relatively homogeneous populations. In Germany, for example, Africans and Turks have taken up residence where mostly only native-born Germans have lived.

Social changes such as these may bring many positive benefits along with the stress. Nevertheless, it seems clear that each new wave of hospice programs will begin in a somewhat different context and face a different configuration of needs, challenges, and resources. Accordingly, it might be disastrous for hospice leaders to focus so intently on their own particular daily responsibilities that they ignore the larger changes that could endanger their efforts. Hospice leaders could contribute much to academic disciplines such as sociology, anthropology, and psychology and, in turn, enhance their understanding of the forces that will affect palliative care programs in the years ahead.

3. Intrinsic changes are also taking place in world population. More people are living to advanced ages. Along with this near-universal trend, there are also many local changes in population structure that result in different configurations of residents within a household and different ratios of workers to dependent people (children, disabled, and aged). There are positive facets to these changes, e.g., the experience and wisdom of elders within a society. There are also additional burdens and constraints, however, as in the increasing age of the primary family caregiver for a terminally ill person. Individual hospice programs throughout the world must find their own solutions to the particular changes that will continue to occur in population structure.

4. The variety of terminal illnesses for which hospice can provide relief has not yet been fully established. As seen particularly in responses to the international survey, there are some marked differences among individual hospices in the type and percentage of terminal conditions that have been under their care, although cancer generally predominates. Some hospices are already dealing extensively with people in the final stages of AIDS-related illness, while others report little or no experience with cases of this kind. Conspicuously, but not surprisingly, people whose terminal illness is related to cardiovascular failure are very seldom partici-

pants in hospice programs. We do not yet know the full potential of palliative care programs for comforting patients whose conditions depart significantly from the "model dying trajectory" of terminal cancer. This means we also do not yet know what conditions might require quite a different approach to care and comfort than any of the models currently in existence. Furthermore, we also do not know what rare or new terminal conditions might appear at any time. It would be useless to speculate here on the forms these conditions might take, but it would also be naive to suppose that from this point on the world will be spared new threats to life and, perhaps, new horrors. Hospice personnel in every locale and at every level might be well advised to keep themselves informed on epidemiological and sociotechnological changes that could confront them with major new challenges to palliative care skills and resources.

5. "Bureaucratic creep" is the term that might be given to a challenge that hospice programs face from the inside as well as the outside. Hospice pioneers generally have had to wrestle with existing bureaucracies to create an opening for their programs and obtain some measure of financial support. There have been a few glittering exceptions (such as the quick and positive response of the government in Saudi Arabia), but most often the bureaucracy has neglected or opposed early hospice efforts by behaving, well, bureaucratically!

The irony of hospice success has not been lost on many of the pioneers, who realize that this achievement has required a certain degree of bureaucratization of their own agencies. Few if any would argue against such basic bureaucratic procedures as financial accountability, and few if any would argue that hospice, alone of all social institutions, should not be subject to any regulations. There is some danger, however, that some hospice programs may become too routinized and too rigid as they accommodate themselves to regulations and other constraints. Even greater is the danger that the focus might shift—imperceptibly at first, but then decisively—away from the original humanitarian mission to "the agency for the agency's sake." This is what is meant here by "bureaucratic creep." No organization is entirely immune to this threat, so here is one more challenge that hospice leaders will need to cope with on a continuing basis.

## CONCLUDING THOUGHT

Hospice care has come a long way in a short time. It has also come a long way from its origins in the United Kingdom (where the practice of palliative care continues to evolve). No matter what area of the globe, no matter what languages are spoken, no matter what level of technological development, the communities of the world have welcomed hospice concepts and practice once they have seen them in action. Many thousands of people have lived in greater comfort and security as their lives came to an end, and many families have participated in this process and come away with a greater sense of accomplishment and serenity.

But there is something more. Hospice seems to be accomplishing even more than its primary mission. Hospice is providing the opportunity for people to rediscover their common humanity. Hospice is providing the opportunity for people to rediscover their ability to provide comfort to each other under the most trying circumstances. Hospice is providing the opportunity for all the people of all the nations in the world to feel again their faith, their compassion, their humanity. May this process so continue.

# Appendix: Regional Data

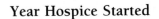

Year Hospice Started

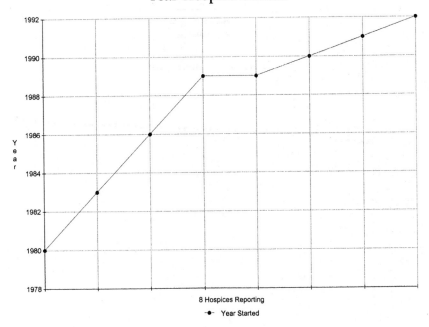

FIGURE 3-1b  Africa

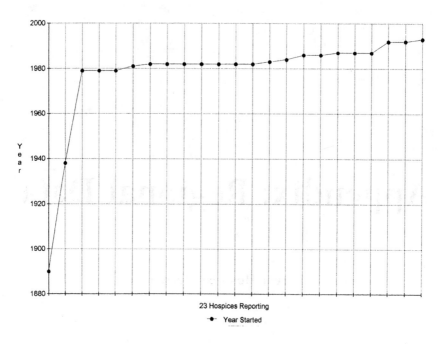

23 Hospices Reporting

-•- Year Started

FIGURE 3-1c  Australasia

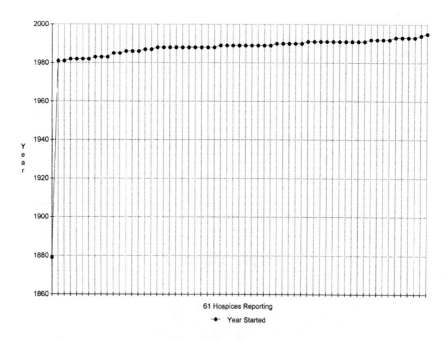

61 Hospices Reporting

-•- Year Started

FIGURE 3-1d  Europe

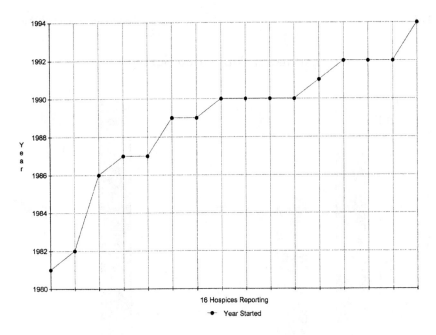

FIGURE 3-1e  Far East and Southeast Asia

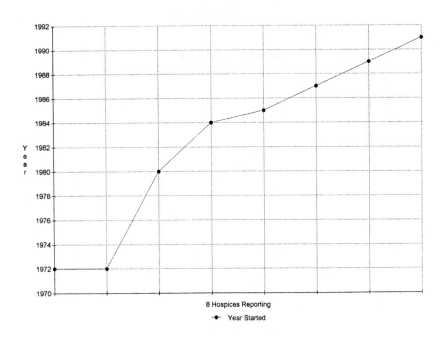

FIGURE 3-1f  South America

# Estimated Population Served

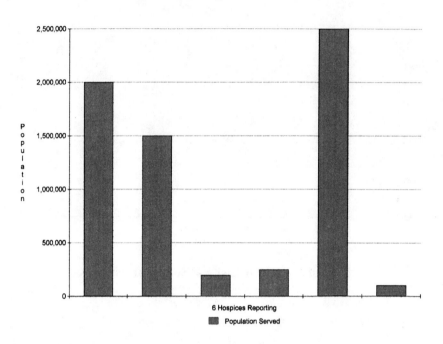

FIGURE 3-2b  Africa

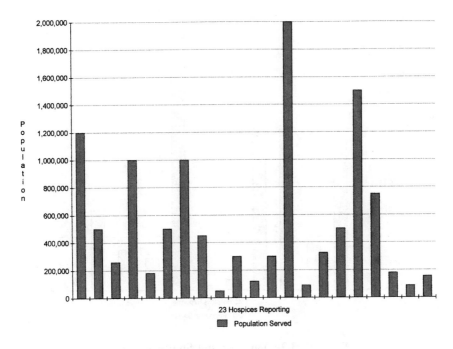

FIGURE 3-2c  Australasia

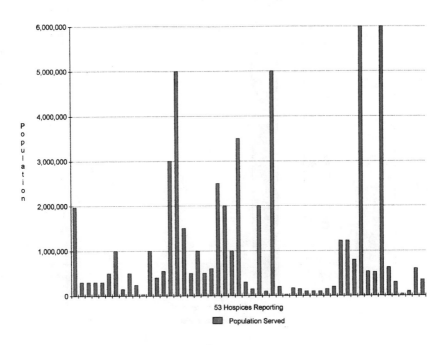

FIGURE 3-2d  Europe

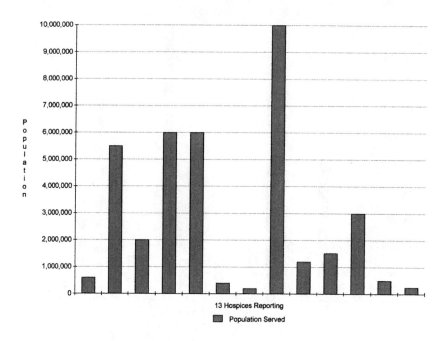

FIGURE 3-2e  Far East and Southeast Asia

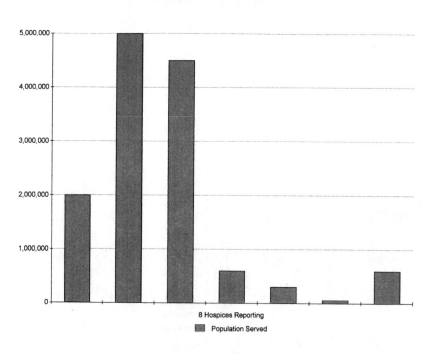

FIGURE 3-2f  South America

## Clients Served Per Year

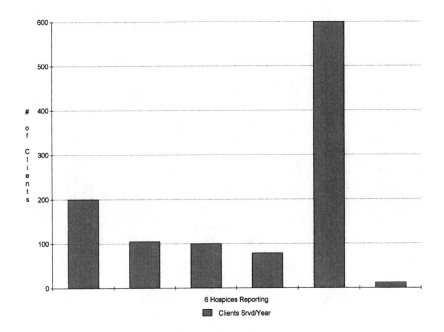

FIGURE 3-3b  Africa

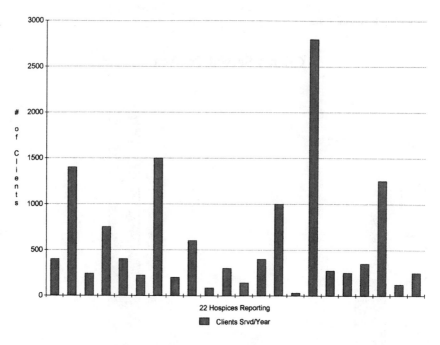

FIGURE 3-3c  Australasia

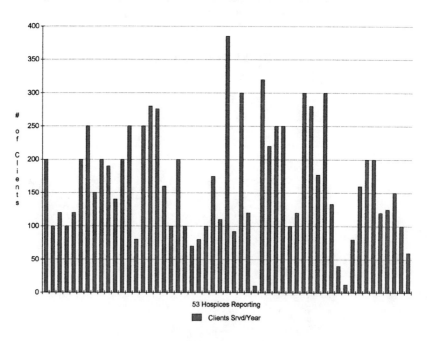

FIGURE 3-3d  Europe

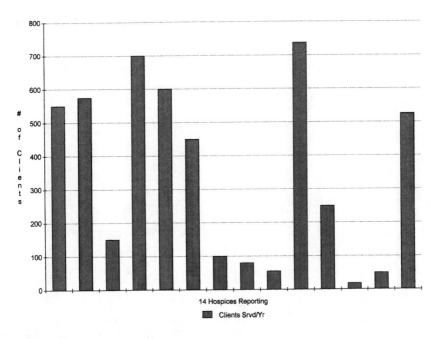

FIGURE 3-3e  Far East and Southeast Asia

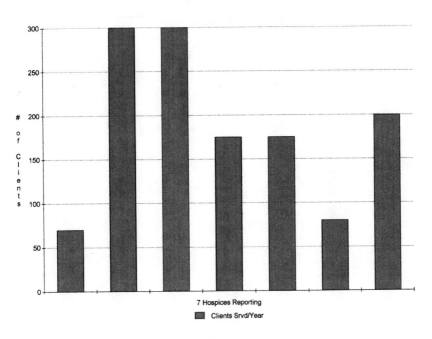

FIGURE 3-3f  South America

# Age of Clients

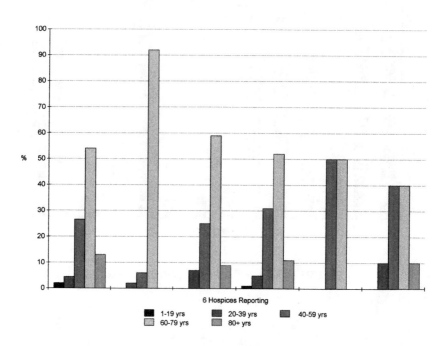

FIGURE 3-4b  Africa

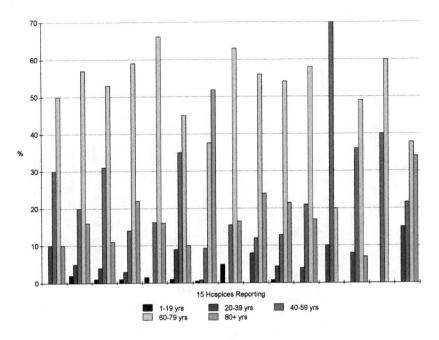

FIGURE 3-4c  Australasia

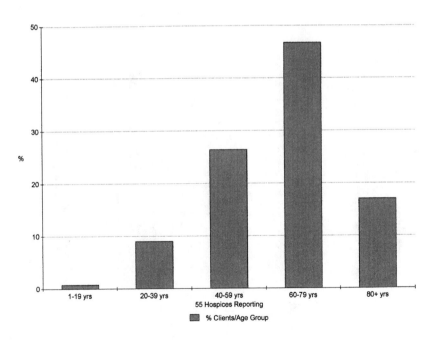

FIGURE 3-4d  Europe

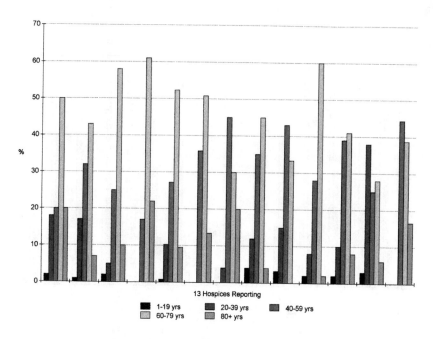

FIGURE 3-4e  Far East and Southeast Asia

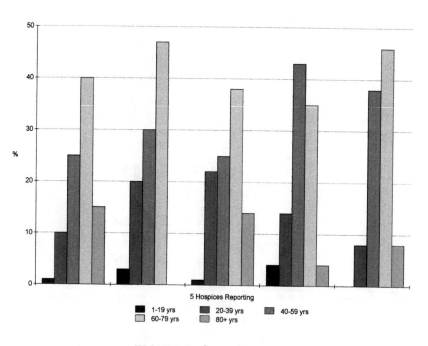

FIGURE 3-4f  South America

# Ratio of Females to Males

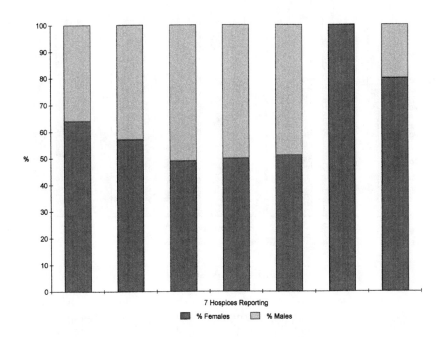

FIGURE 3-5b  Africa

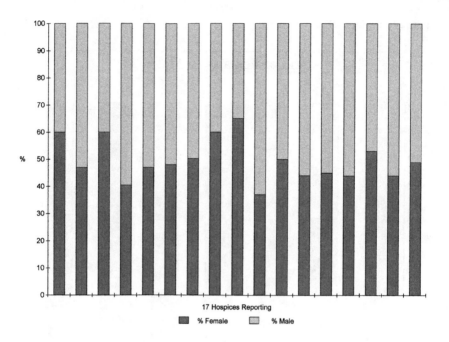

FIGURE 3-5c  Australasia

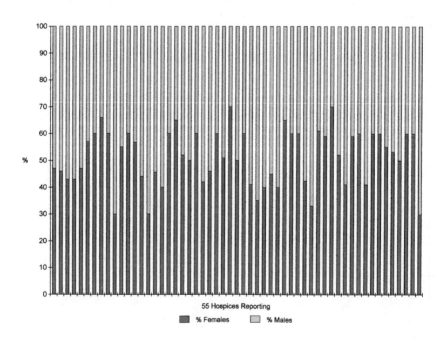

FIGURE 3-5d  Europe

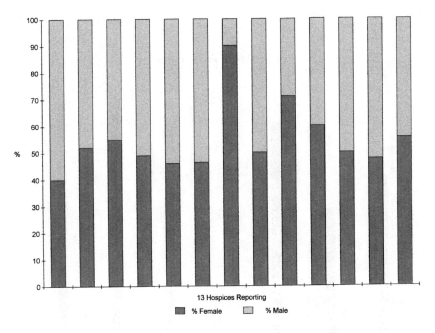

FIGURE 3-5e  Far East and Southeast Asia

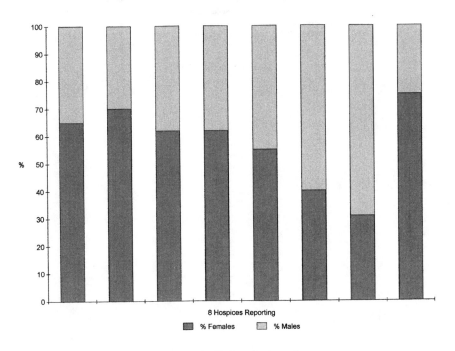

FIGURE 3-5f  South America

## Location of Services

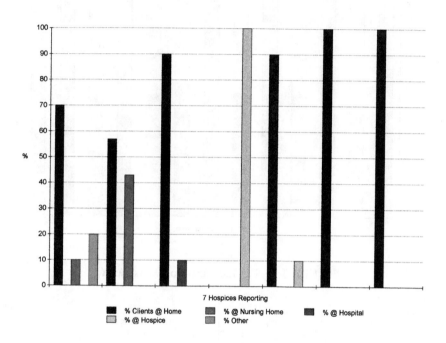

7 Hospices Reporting

| ■ % Clients @ Home | ■ % @ Nursing Home | ■ % @ Hospital |
| □ % @ Hospice | ■ % Other | |

**FIGURE 3-6b  Africa**

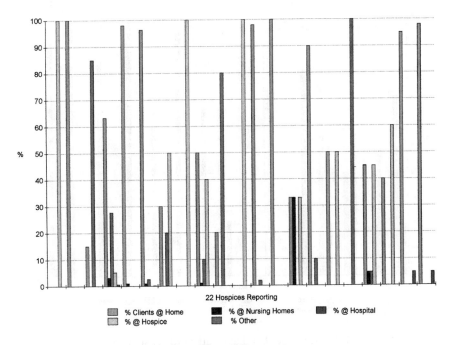

% Clients @ Home   % @ Nursing Homes   % @ Hospital
% @ Hospice   % Other

FIGURE 3-6c  Australasia

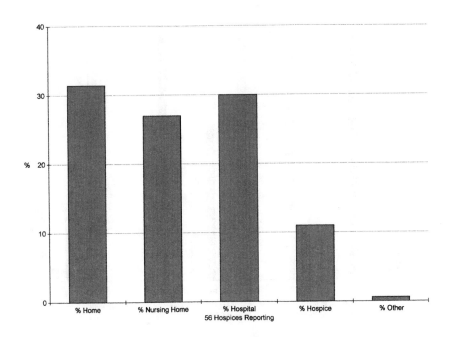

56 Hospices Reporting

% Home   % Nursing Home   % Hospital   % Hospice   % Other

FIGURE 3-6d  Europe

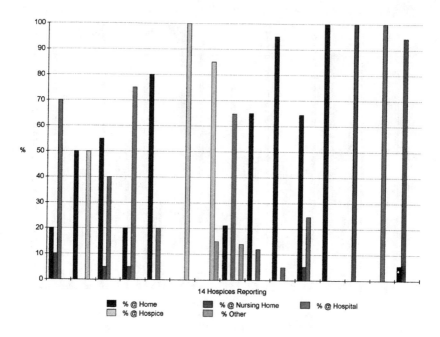

**FIGURE 3-6e  Far East and Southeast Asia**

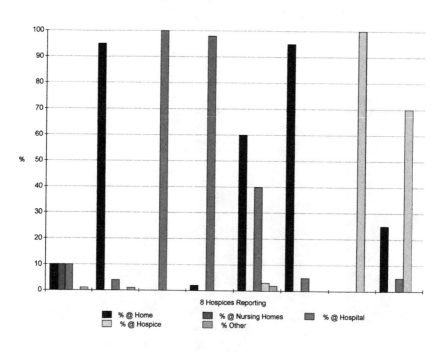

**FIGURE 3-6f  South America**

# Sources of Funding

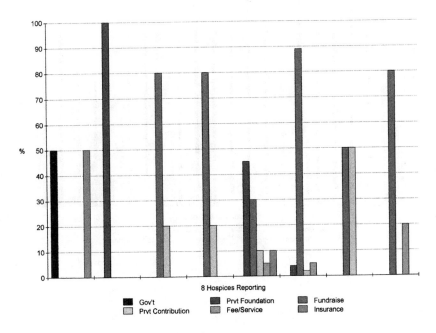

8 Hospices Reporting

■ Gov't                ■ Prvt Foundation        ■ Fundraise
□ Prvt Contribution    ■ Fee/Service            ■ Insurance

FIGURE 3-7b  Africa

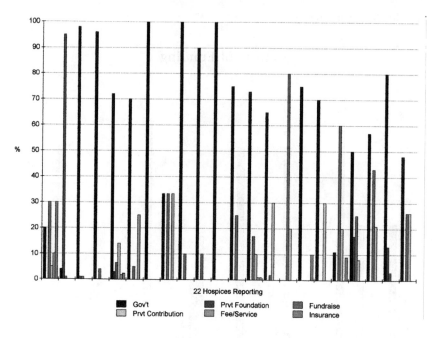

FIGURE 3-7c Australasia

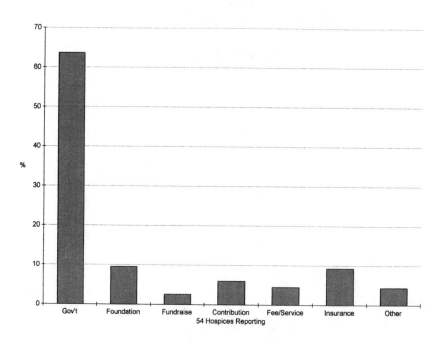

FIGURE 3-7d Europe

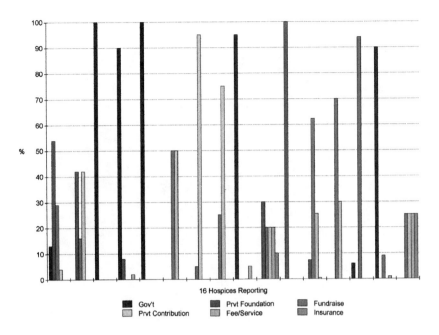

FIGURE 3-7e  Far East and Southeast Asia

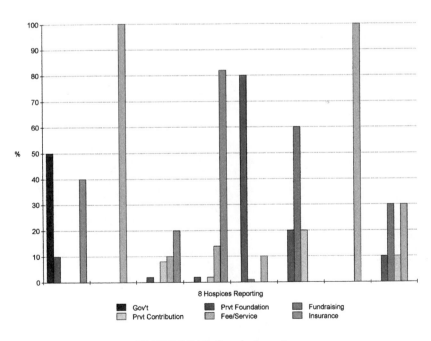

FIGURE 3-7f  South America

# Index

Acquired immunodeficiency syndrome
(AIDS), impact of
on program in Bermuda, 69–70
on program in South Africa, 48–49
on program in United States, 110
Age, in international hospice survey, 28–
31, 30f
AIDS. *See* Acquired immunodeficiency
syndrome (AIDS)
Al-Malath Foundation for Humanistic
Care, 242–253. *See also* Jordan,
hospice programs in
Analgesic ladder, of World Health
Organization, 16–17, 202–203
Apartheid, provision of hospice services
during, 47
Architectural design, of hospice facilities,
135
Assisted suicide
and hospice care, 111–112
public policy on, 11

Bereavement care
in program in France, 138
in program in South Africa, 44–45
Bermuda, hospice programs in, 61–72
accomplishments of, 70
development of, 61–64
funding of, 65–67
goals of, 71
impact of AIDS on, 69–70
management of, 67–68

nursing care in, 68–69
office space for, 65
patient financial assistance in, 66
recommendations by, 71
staffing of, 66
transportation in, 69
Bureaucracy, 267
Bureaucratic creep, 271

Canada, hospice programs in, 73–84
accomplishments of, 84
consultation with St. Christopher's
Hospice by, 75–76
development of, 73–75, 77–78
funding of, 81–82
goals of, 83–84
growth of, 83
influence on French programs, 131
palliative care before, 73–74
resistance to, 79–81
volunteers in, 82–83
Cancer, distribution of, by site, in
international hospice survey, 32
Cancer pain. *See* Pain control
Cancer Relief India, 213
Caregivers, hospice programs for persons
without, 110
Care planning conferences. *See also*
Multidisciplinary collaboration
psychological consultation for, 140
Catchment areas, size of, in international
hospice survey, 26–27, 27f

**⑤** *Springer Publishing Company*

# Spirituality in Nursing
## From Traditional to New Age
**Barbara Stevens Barnum,** RN, PhD, FAAN

In this thoughtful examination of
the reemergence of spirituality as
an important factor in nursing
practice, the author traces nursing's
involvement with spirituality from
its historical ties with religion to the
current interest in alternative health
methods. New nursing theories that
involve spirituality, such as those of
Dossey, Newman, and Watson are
described. And nursing trends are
put in the larger context of trends in
society and other disciplines, such as psychology, physics,
and philosophy.

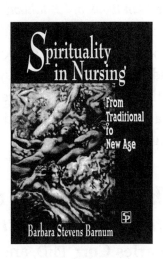

*Contents:*
- Spirituality in Nursing: Origins, Development, Overview
- Spirituality and Nursing's History
- Spirituality as a Component in Nursing Theory
- Developmental Theories: Is There a Spiritual Phase?
- Spirituality and the Emerging Paradigm
- Nursing Theorists in the New Paradigm
- Nursing and Healing
- Spirituality and Ethics: A Contrast in Forms
- Ethics and Philosophy
- Spirituality and the Mind
- Spirituality, Disease, and Death
- Spirituality and Religion
- Spiritual Therapeutics

*1995  176pp  0-8261-9180-0  hardcover*

536 Broadway, New York, NY 10012-3955 • (212) 431-4370 • Fax (212) 941-7842

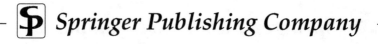

# Ⓢ *Springer Publishing Company*

# Grief Counseling and
# Grief Therapy, Second Edition
## *A Handbook for the*
## *Mental Health Practitioner*
### J. William Worden, PhD

This best-selling text includes authoritative material on AIDS and bereavement, grief and the elderly, grief counseling groups, and a greatly expanded bibliography.

*"I like Worden's sensitive, insightful view of special losses, particularly his discussion of SIDS deaths and his discussion of AIDS....Worden provides a training model for grief counseling. The instructions are clear on how to structure the training, and Worden offers several vignettes for role-playing and group interaction."*
—Journal of Palliative Care

*"...well organized, concrete in its detail, emotionally stirring in its use of language and concise in its superb review of the current state of knowledge..."*
—Journal of Psychology & Theology

*Partial Contents:*

Attachment, Loss and the Tasks of Mourning • Normal Grief Reactions: Uncomplicated Mourning • Grief Counseling: Facilitating Uncomplicated Grief • Abnormal Grief Reactions: Complicated Mourning • Grief Therapy: Resolving Pathological Grief • Grieving Special Types of Losses • Grief and Family Systems • The Counselor's Own Grief • Training for Grief Counseling

*Behavioral Science Book Service Selection*
*1991   200pp   0-8261-4161-7   hardcover*

536 Broadway, New York, NY 10012-3955 • (212) 431-4370 • Fax (212) 941-7842

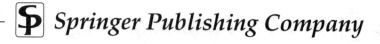
# *Springer Publishing Company*

# *Suicide and Agimg*
### Jane L. Pearson, PhD
### Yeates Conwell, MD, Editors

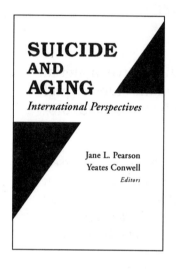

**SUICIDE AND AGING**
*International Perspectives*

Jane L. Pearson
Yeates Conwell
*Editors*

Based on a special issue of *International Psychogeriatrics*, this volume explores the risk factors and clinical profiles of late-life suicide in the hope of gaining a better understanding of this phenomenon. Renowned international researchers examine how the aging process, cultural factors, cohort effects, personality, medical disorders, and the concept of an individual's life course trajectory may contribute to the incidence of suicide. This book is valuable for professionals, educators, and graduate students in the social and health sciences, including psychology, psychiatry, gerontology, geriatrics, nursing, and sociology.

### Partial Contents:

- Suicide and Aging I: Patterns of Psychiatric Diagnosis, *Y. Conwell and D. Brent*

- Suicide and Aging II: The Psychobiological Interface, *Y. Conwell, et al.*

- Suicide, Life Course, and Life Story, *B.J. Cohler and M.J. Jenuwine*

- Reflections on Culutral Influences on Aging and Old-Age Suicide in Germany, *R. Schmitz-Schezer*

- Suicide in Later Life in Japan: Urban and Rural Differences, *N. Watanabe, et al.*

- Suicide in the Elderly: The United Kingdom Perspective, *M.S. Dennis and J. Lindesay*

- Mental Disorders in Elderly Suicide, *M.M. Henriksson, et al.*

*1996    256pp    0-8261-9370-6    hardcover*

536 Broadway, New York, NY 10012-3955 • (212) 431-4370 • Fax (212) 941-7842